The Five-Factors of Fitness For Him
The Simple Evidence-Based Way to Lose Fat and Keep it off

By

William E. Cecrle

For Sunshine: You are the light of my life!

To Bobby: Thanks for the idea!

To Dad and Mom: Thanks for the inspiration!

Table of Contents

Introduction

In this brief story, I present you with a great deal of what I have learned from my studies in occupational therapy, theology, nutrition, and exercise science about how people best lose fat and make permanent lifestyle changes.

By "best," I mean how people make connections to the truths of fat loss, use those connections to produce results, and either get in the best "shape" of their lives or know why they have not!

This allegory, *The Five Factors of Fitness*, is a synthesis of what many wise people have taught me and what I have learned myself over 15 years of training and educating thousands of people. I recognize these sources of wisdom. I also recognize that we are sources of wisdom concerning ourselves and that we are the experts about ourselves. The purpose of this allegory is to provide a paradigmatic structure wherein we can exercise that wisdom and successfully change for the better.

I trust, therefore, that you will take the practical knowledge you gain from this book and use it in your daily life. For as it has been so aptly noted, "Knowledge is not power, *applied* knowledge is power!"

I hope that you enjoy *applying* what you learn from *The Five Factors of Fitness* and that, as a result, you live a healthier, happier and more satisfying life.

Bill Cecrle, BA, MA, NASM, MOTR/L

The Five Factors of Fitness

Prologue

Once there was a young man who wanted to break the bondage of yo-yo dieting, cut through the clutter of T.V. infomercials, and gain control of his body and health. He sought help from his doctors, who were very knowledgeable about diseases, drugs, and surgeries. The doctors were good people who were highly educated (some of the smartest people he had ever met) and they were genuine about wanting to help him. He was disappointed to hear that they did not receive any formal education concerning nutrition. Regardless, he spent a couple years trying to use this approach. These people were the best our society had to offer, right? But these methods didn't seem to answer his questions and he didn't change his body or his life. His body aging and frustration mounting, he abandoned this approach and turned to the T.V. gurus and their promises of "six-pack abs", easy weight loss, and too-good-to-be-true supplements—which they were! These people made many promises that turned out to be either completely false or half-truths. The driving factor for them seemed to be making money, not helping him. After trying 'just one more pill' he knew that the answers he sought would not be found with them. In his heart he knew the answer could not have been that easy. So, once again he moved on to find the answers to a healthy and a beautiful body.

On a Facebook posting discussing fitness, the young man was told that he needed to "go natural" and everything would fall into place. He tried this too and had the same results as before—maybe a little success, then back to where he started or worse.

He was in his 30's now and a feeling of hopelessness wrapped itself around him. Maybe he didn't have the genetics to be fit? Maybe his quest had been an open but futile rebellion against who he was? Maybe it was time to accept the inevitable—he would always have a little bit of a gut, not like his body, and be at higher risk for certain health issues. He was telling this to his coworkers at lunch when one of them said,

"Brother, don't do that! You can do it—anyone can! You just need to master the Five Factors of Fitness and you will get what you want."

The man replied, "That's easy for you to say, you are in good shape!"

His coworker looked him squarely in the eye and said, "Exactly. But I wasn't always this way. If you're serious about change, call this guy's number and he'll help." He pulled out his cell phone, wrote a number on a napkin, and slid it towards the man. Slightly embarrassed the man ignored it until lunch was over and everyone was leaving—then he grabbed the napkin and put it into his purse. He would do whatever it took; besides what would it hurt to give it one more try?

And so after work he called the number...

"The Five Factors of Fitness"

The voice on the phone was gentle and articulate, not the drill-sergeant gruffness he had expected. After he introduced himself, the voice on the other end of the phone line said he was a Fitness and Health Trainer and he asked the simple question, "What do you want?"

To which he responded, "To lose weight."

"No, you don't." Was the quick, matter-of-fact answer.

He was silent, taken aback. Who was he? Thinking he knows me better than myself?

As he thought this the voice continued, "I was like you once—on a journey to understand myself, my body, and to know how best to make it the way I wanted it to be."

To his surprise instead of lambasting the trainer for arrogance when he opened his mouth he said, "That's right!"

The voice continued, "What you want is to know how to get a healthy, good-looking body and keep it that way."

He was nodding his head yes as it continued, "You want to be a Master of the Five Factors of Fitness!"

He realized he had been nodding his head unconsciously when the trainer couldn't see it. "A what?"

"A Master of the Five Factors of Fitness. Someone who understands the five parts of health and fitness and how to apply them to his own body. Someone who wants to control their body and life instead of being controlled by food, fatigue, and fads!"

The man was on his feet now saying, "Yes! That's exactly what I want!"

There was silence on the other side of the phone for what seemed an eternity. Then the voice said, "It will cost you. Are you prepared for that?"

His smile faltered and his shoulders slumped just a little. Oh no, this was starting to sound just like his attempt through the T.V. infomercials!

The voice continued, "It is a service for a fee; but if you are like I was, and all the others I have helped, it will be the cost of time and energy that will be the most challenging part for you. That and the discipline!"

"I can be disciplined!" The man retorted.

"Good. You will need to be. I will commit to you if you commit to me and do everything I ask of you." He affirmed that he would and the trainer gave him a time and place for them to meet.

Factor One

Nutrition

(or Hand-to-Mouth Disease)

When the man met the trainer he was what he had expected; it appeared he practiced what he preached. As he entered the clinic the trainer confidently approached him and gave him a hearty handshake.

"Let's get down to business." The trainer said as he motioned to a set of chairs and round table. First he took a series of measurements and the young man's body-fat percentage was calculated. The trainer showed him a chart that indicated he was in the highest category of body-fat and told him of all the health-related diseases he was at risk of developing.

"Wait a minute!" He stopped the trainer. "I can't be in the *worst* group; I know all kinds of people that are way heavier than I am! I am one of the smaller people I know!"

The trainer patiently listened as he described his friends and family, all of whom he described as much heavier than himself. When he stopped the trainer said, "I believe that everything you said is true; but that does not make what we found today false. You see; we are all creatures of relativity. We see, experience, and interpret the world through its relation to us. Most of the people around you probably are heavier and fatter than you. But that only makes it *seem* that you are healthy when in reality you are only less heavy and fat! It is a common mistake most of us make—myself included from time to time. We need to rely on the objective scientific measures not the subjective observations to guide us, okay?"

He quickly processed and understood what the trainer said and knew it to be true then agreed with him.

"Moving forward we will measure you with your body weight, fat mass percentage, and circumference measurements. Only with the combination of these three biometrics can we truly understand what is happening to your body. A person can lose weight, but it all can be fat-free mass, and he is becoming less healthy and looking worse. Or a person can *gain* weight and *lose* fat, improving his health and looking better. The only way to know for certain is for these assessments to be performed!"

The next hour was a grueling question/answer session where topics from the most mundane to the most personal were discussed. Mentally fatigued from the interview he almost missed that the trainer was pausing for yet another answer.

"Yes. I am ready for this." He insisted.

The trainer smiled. "Good. Then know this: my philosophy of training is an educational one. I will not just tell you what to do, but why you need to do it and why it works. Everything I teach you is backed by the best evidence research has given us so far coupled with my thousands of hours of experience. You will be in the best shape of your life or you will know why you are not! I will not always be around to help you so it is important that you learn these lessons. And yes, there will be a test!" He paused, looking at the young man's slumped shoulders and glazed eyes. "You look like you have had enough for the day. Let's start next time with the first Factor—Nutrition. Bring me a food journal for the three days prior to our session; make sure to record *everything* that goes into your mouth!"

The young man took his leave, tired but excited!

The next time he entered the clinic the trainer was seated behind the desk, which was covered in food! It looked like a continuum of bad food to good food with the left side of the table piled with chips, cookies, doughnuts, and bacon; the middle filled with cheeses, breads, pasta, and meats; and the right side of the table piled with fresh vegetables and fruits. The man walked forward smiling, wondering what exactly this was all about.

As the young man neared the table the trainer spread his arms saying, "Welcome to Nutrition 101!" The man sat at his chair noticing that the food was plastic and rubber. He placed his homework on the desk.

Smiling, the trainer acknowledged it and said, "Which of these foods can prevent you from achieving your goal?"

The man carefully thought of all the diets he had tried (No Carb, High Carb, No Fat, Only Fruit, Only "Natural", and Vegan) and shrugged. "The only thing I can say for sure is that these on the left are bad."

The trainer was just sitting there looking at him. "This next part is *very* important for you to know. Regarding fat loss, there really are not any foods that will keep you from success. You look surprised! And you should; we constantly hear about diets and the things we can't have! The truth is that it is *not* about what you have but about how *much* you have! This goes back to physics. Yes, you will be learning a couple of the principles of physics so that you are able to understand and control your body! The first one is called the First Law of Thermodynamics[1]. It is called a 'law' because it is *always* true."

---

[1] Underlined words are defined with examples in the Glossary of the book.

The man had begun to look intimidated since "physics" was mentioned, so the trainer softened his tone. "Listen, you already know some of this physics stuff! For example, what happens when you step off a cliff?"

"You fall." He said.

"How about a building?'

""You fall."

"A curb?"

"You fall."

The trainer grinned, "That's right! You fall and we know because of the *Law* of Gravity that you will always be pulled towards the center of the Earth if there is nothing beneath you! That's the Law of Gravity: Physics! The First Law of Thermodynamics states that energy is neither created nor destroyed, only converted into another form of energy. When we apply that Law to our bodies it says that when we consume (through eating and drinking) energy (calories) that energy has only two choices. One, be converted into energy and used or to become stored energy—which we store where?"

The man patted his gut.

The trainer nodded. "Yep! That's where it goes on you. The point is that regardless of the type of food you eat if you consume more calories than you use then your body *must* store them. They cannot just 'go away'! That's a Law of Physics applied to your body! No ifs, ands, or buts about it; if you consume excess, it gets stored as fat and if you don't consume enough…"

A sign of understanding flashed through the man's eyes, "Your body uses fat to make up the difference?!"

"Exactly!" The trainer said noticing a slight frown cross the man's face. He was processing it all so he waited.

"But aren't carbs bad for you and make you gain weight?"

The trainer nodded, "Yes and no. No, they are *not* bad for you; your body needs them to be healthy! It only *feels* like they are bad because they help you retain water—which is super important for your health! When you cut out carbs you lose a bunch of weight but it is mostly water-weight—which you don't want to lose! Then when a person reintroduces carbs the water weight rushes back on and that person says 'Aha! Carbs are bad!' But really it is a slight-of-hand shell-game that is bad for your health. Does that make sense?"

He saw that the man was still confused so he switched approaches, "Your body is like a bank account. Calories are the currency we use at this bank; they are like dollars. When you asked about carbs that was like asking about a smaller unit of the dollar, say a nickel. We call things like carbs 'Macronutrients' because they are the large building blocks of nutrition. There are 5 major macronutrients we will learn about and use or avoid during our time together. He pulled out a laminated sheet that read:

---

1 gram of fat= 9 calories
1 gram of alcohol=7 calories
1 gram of carbohydrate=4 calories
1 gram of protein =4 calories
1 gram of water=0 calories

"These 5 macronutrients (he slid his finger down the sheet pointing to each line: fat, alcohol, carbs, proteins, and water) are essential to understand because they make up everything we consume! Here's the kicker—they all have different values of energy per unit of mass. Fats have 9 calories per gram—which is the most calorically expensive! This is why 20-30 years ago the diet fads were all—'You are what you eat; don't eat fat or you will be fat.' It is a half-truth. Fats have a disproportionately high amount of calories but eating fat doesn't make you fat; eating too many calories is what makes you fat! Alcohol is the next most expensive macronutrient—it has 7 calories per gram; however, there is virtually no nutritional value with these calories. They have an extremely limited and low number of *micro*nutrients. These are the building blocks of *macro*nutrients and we will talk about them later when we discuss supplementation. The next most expensive are carbs and proteins, these both have 4 calories per gram. So you see, carbs are twice as 'good' as fats and the same as proteins! Again, I like to think of it as an account at a bank. When you deposit a check into your account the balance only reflects the dollar amount; they don't say you have X dollar bills, X quarters, X dimes, X nickels, and X pennies. They simply record and report it in dollars and fractions of dollars. Your body-fat is the same. If you are 500 calories over your expenditure for that 24 hour period then your body will store it as fat the same if it came from proteins, carbs, or fats!"

"So all these diets and books about no/low carb, high protein, or low fat…"

"They are gimmicks playing off half-truths! Their purpose is to make money whether or not they are being accurate. I believe and hope that most *do* want to help people too but that they are not grounded in an evidence-based approach."

"What's that?" The man interjected.

"It is an approach that takes more than simple observation, experience, and reason to make decisions on how to help people. It means taking into account the best scientific data that has been published and synthesizing it with personal experience to find the best answer. Carbs seem to make you gain fat until you look at the scientific evidence! Then you know it is the calories, not carbs that does it! What I am going to teach you is based off the best evidence!"

The man's eyes lit up again, "That's what I want!"

"Good, let's go back and talk about the macronutrients. Although they have the same effect on your body-fat they are composed of different micronutrients, which support different physiological functions within the body. There are three things I want you to remember about the macronutrients. First, they help determine your health. Too much or too little of any macronutrients is not healthy for you. There are things that only proteins, carbs, or fats can do for you—the others can't do it! Second, they have a strong influence on or satiety, or your feeling of fullness and satisfaction after eating. Finally, they play an integral role in your body's ability to regulate your energy levels."

"What type of things do they do different?" He asked.

"Carbohydrates are the major source of energy for the body because they are the quickest to turn into blood sugar, or glucose; this is because they are just a different form of sugar. They are the preferred fuel for basic body functions like breathing and activities like walking. Carbohydrates are best understood as three distinct categories: sugars, starches, and fiber. The first two are broken down and used as energy and the third is neither digested nor absorbed. High fiber foods do two things to help us lose fat. First, they do not provide many calories because they are not broken-down and absorbed. Second, they give more volume to your stomach contents, which makes you feel fuller. Here is one reason to avoid refined foods and grains. The refining process removes fiber and many other nutrients to give the food a finer texture and longer shelf life. Some of these are 'enriched' to put back in some of those micronutrients (typically Iron and B vitamins) but they are never as filling or nutritious as they once were!

Fats are a great source of long-lasting energy for the body and they transport fat-soluble vitamins through the blood and into cells. Fat-soluble vitamins can only survive and gain access into certain cells by 'piggy-backing' on fats because those cells have a kind of chemical lock that only fats have the keys to fit. If there are no fats then those cells cannot let in the micronutrients! Examples of these are vitamins like A, D, E, and K. Fats can be broken down into three basic categories too. There are Trans fats, which should be avoided at all costs and are by far the least healthy of all fats; Saturated fats, which are less damaging to your health but still not the best type of fat to consume; and finally there are unsaturated fats, which have the 'good' cholesterol and are better for your health.[2] Remember, in terms of fat loss there is no difference but in terms of your health there is a huge one! Fats are also important because they transport flavor and give texture to foods. Both of these are extremely important to satiety, which we will discuss in a little while."

The trainer handed him a card that read:

Macronutrients:

Proteins, Carbs, Fats, Alcohol, Water

1. Keep you healthy
2. Keep you satisfied
3. Keep you energetic

---

[2] www.american heart.org

As he read it the trainer continued, "Here is where a half-truth has infused itself into popular culture regarding food. You were *kinda* correct when you said the left side of the table was full of bad foods. Most of those foods are high on the Glycemic Index."

He pulled out a paper and pen, and then drew a chart on it.

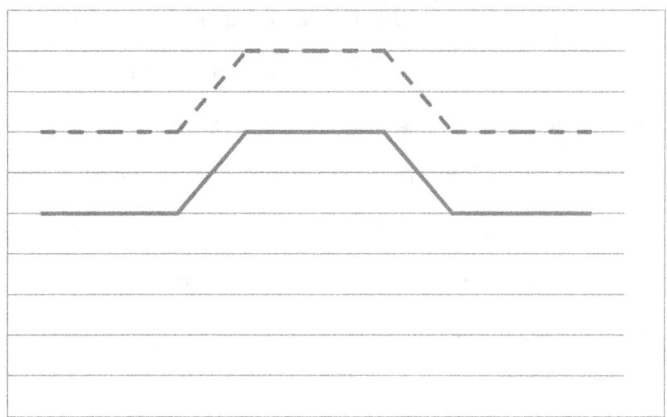

"Going up the X-axis is the level of blood sugar, or glucose, and across the Y-axis is time. This solid line is your glucose. Food and drinks with calories eventually are converted into glucose so that your body can use it. Do you know what regulates our glucose?"

He nodded excitedly, "Yes, insulin!" I have a diabetic father!"

"Good job—that's right! Insulin is a very powerful hormone and its job is to not allow glucose levels to rise too high or to fall too low otherwise we have very serious health problems! So, this dashed line is your insulin and it keeps your glucose in check—constantly shuttling glucose from cells into your bloodstream and from your bloodstream into your cells depending on your needs. Here is where your nutrition comes into play. When you eat foods high on the Glycemic Index they quickly turn into glucose."

He was drawing another graph as he spoke. "That is the spike you see on this graph. This freaks your insulin out and it says 'Oh crap, we're going to die!' and it over regulates— shuttling too much glucose into cells (the dashed spike).

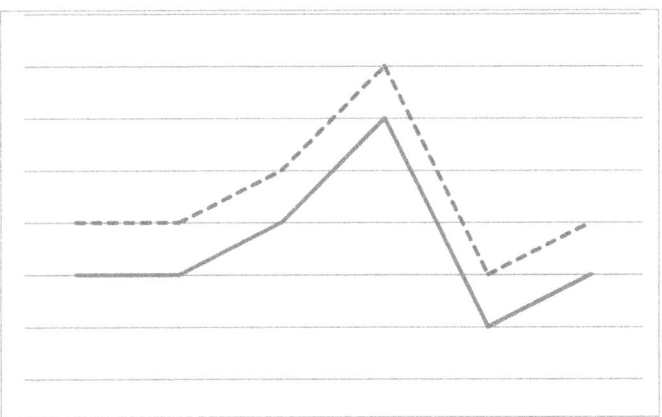

Well at that point you have a huge dip in your blood sugar and you feel that sluggish 'I need a nap' feeling. Slowly your insulin backs off and your glucose rises back up to the pre-meal level. In the meantime, most people have tried to pick back up by eating or drinking something sugary again to re-spike their insulin, which is real hard on your body in many ways."

"I see co-workers do that all the time at work! After lunch they have a candy bar then an hour later they have a Pepsi or Coke, then they snack on candy until work is over!"

"Exactly. What you will learn is that you have a specific ratio of carbohydrates, proteins, and fats that *you* need to be healthy, satisfied and energetic. Many successful weight losers need almost 30% of their food to come from fats and some need only 15%.[3] Everyone is different. I have clients who have needed as much as 75% of their food to come from carbohydrates and some people as low as 45%!"

"Why so different?"

"Well, I don't know for certain but we are all individuals and our bodies reflect that. I remember in gross anatomy we had twelve cadavers in our lab and when we were not dissecting we could go look at other groups' cadavers. This gave me a great appreciation for just how different we all are. Ten of the twelve cadavers would be textbook but one was usually a little different and one was often significantly different. On a smaller scale, with our biochemistry, it is the same thing. Some bodies work best with more of the micronutrients in carbs, other best with more of the micronutrients in fats. Proteins stay consistent at around a quarter of calories consumed. About 85% of my clients over the years have fallen into a ratio of 60% carbs, 20% proteins, and 20% fats. The information we gathered last session puts you into that category too. There are no hard and fast rules for determining these so we will have to observe your changes and make adjustments as needed.[4] Your body composition, sex, age, and activity level put you at a daily caloric need of 1,750 per day. These are just 'best-guesses' based off algorithms so we will monitor your body composition and make adjustments as needed."

"So the half-truth is that the foods are not bad for fat loss, just your health?"

The trainer weighed his response before answering. "Well, that is almost the whole truth. The part that you did not say is really a nuance; it is that although those foods don't make

---

[3] Phelan S, Wyatt HR, Hill JO, et al. *Obesity*. 2006; 14:710-716.
[4] Irwin, T. New Dietary Guidelines from the American Diabetes Association. *Diabetes Care*. 2002;25:1262-1263.

you fat because of *what* they are they do make most people fat because of *how* they make people feel. Food engineers construct those foods to give us the most pleasure possible when we eat them. This makes us crave more food and more foods that are high in calories but low in nutrients. This makes us over-consume calories and increase body-fat."

The man frowned, "If the foods are high in calories why doesn't our body tell us to stop eating?

"That's a great question! Unfortunately, the answer is really complex, individualized, and we are not certain that we fully understand it. There are some things that we know for certain.

Hunger and satiety is a complex interplay between a person's physiology and psychology. We already discussed one of the physiological factors of hunger when we discussed the need for that certain micronutrients through macronutrient consumption. Have you ever seen kids eat dirt?"

"Oh yes! My nephews did that all the time when they were little!"

"That is a perfect example of a body's physiological needs driving hunger and behavior. Typically those kids are deficient in micronutrients that are minerals. So, their bodies stimulate a craving for dirt because it will deliver those nutrients to the body, even though it is not really 'food'. When we are low in micronutrients our body will try and get us to eat so that we can get those nutrients to stay healthy, fight off diseases, and have energy! This is a huge problem for our society because of the foods we eat. They are low in nutrition and high in calories! We eat them and then still crave food because we have not delivered the nutritional needs of our bodies! Do you remember what I said about alcohol being calorically low value?"

"Yes. You said it had 7 calories per gram but virtually no nutrition!"

"Right! There is almost no nutrition in it so after drinking it our body still wants to consume more to try and get those missing nutrients. The same effect occurs when we eat our 'food products' at a fast food place (or anywhere else) that is high in calories but low in nutrients. One micronutrient that is particularly important for us is fiber. Fiber is a nutrient that causes the feeling of fullness in the stomach and triggers us to stop eating. Very similar to that is a mechanism in the stomach related to the amount of mass consumed. Our stomach stretches as we eat. It is like a balloon that is being inflated. At a certain point it is large enough and there are messages sent that tell us that we are not hungry anymore."

"I had a personal trainer once tell me to drink a bunch of water when I was hungry, it usually worked to keep me from food, but not always."

"That is because hunger is a complex, multifaceted problem! When I was researching my Master's thesis in seminary I found numerous case studies about people who overate because of emotional issues more than physiological ones.[5] One man was hospitalized for malnutrition even though he was morbidly obese and ate around 4,500 calories per day! He was not getting the nutrients with the calories and it was killing him![6]

That brings up the psychological aspect of hunger. Overeating is often a result of trying to gain master and control of oneself. I read this repeatedly in case studies about people struggling with bulimia. Many women feel out of control of their lives and seek that control by binging and purging. I even know of women who have been sexually assaulted and seek

---

[5] Cecrle, W E. *The psychology and spirituality of overeating and obesity in the US.* (2010) Cyclopean Pheonix and William E. Cecrle Publishing. Amazon.com.
[6] Krebs-Smith SM, Guenther PM, Subar AF, Kirkpatrick SI, Dodd KW. Americans do not meet federal dietary recommendations. *Journal of Nutrition* 2010 Oct;140(10):1832-8. Epub 2010 Aug 11.

to de-sexualize themselves by gaining weight. There are many different reasons that psychology can play a role in hunger but the most frequent usually are boredom and stress. Boredom makes us hungry because we are in a low state of arousal and we seek stimulation to arouse ourselves. Stress causes us to eat because we want to replace the mental/emotional pain of the stress with a pleasure, which food delivers. The most easy way to self-medicate and feel better is to eat food to give us a 'pick-me-up'. In fact, some foods also have physiological crossover here! There have been numerous studies on chocolate and how it affects brain chemistry. Researchers have found that chocolate triggers the same chemical pathways in the brain as opiates."[7]

"What are opiates?"

"Opiates are a class of drugs that include Morphine, Heroine, and other mind or mood altering drugs. This tells us that chocolate has the same chemical reward system for our brains as do highly addictive drugs! It is not surprising then that we try to medicate ourselves with foods and that there is at some level a physiological addiction to certain foods too."

"I had no idea! Is that why we shouldn't eat late at night—because we are just feeding an addiction?"

"Heavens no! I am glad you asked that question. This is another one of those half-truth myths floating around the health and fitness scene. Eating late at night will not make you fat…"

The man quickly interjected, "Too many calories will!"

---

[7] Cecrle, W E. *The psychology and spirituality of overeating and obesity in the US.* (2010) Cyclopean Pheonix and William E. Cecrle Publishing. Amazon.com

The trainer nodded approvingly, "Exactly! It does not matter when you eat them, only that you eat fewer than you burned! Our bodies are not like Cinderella's carriage that turns into a pumpkin when the clock strikes midnight! We don't suddenly start processing, storing, and metabolizing nutrients differently! I once had an Emergency Room Nurse Supervisor as a client and she could not eat more than 2 meals on workdays because she was scrubbed in for so many hours in a day. We devised a nutrition plan and menus around two 900-calorie meals on her workdays, one of those meals she ate at midnight! After a year she had lost nearly 40 pounds of fat, showing that the time of day does not matter. Having said that, the truth is that eating late typically is done from boredom or trying to stay awake. When these are the catalyst for eating it almost always is adding calories to a person *past* their daily expenditure. This is a primary reason that late-night television watching is so dangerous for people wanting to lose fat. When we stay up to watch TV past normal day hours we get tired and eat to stay awake! Well, sitting and watching TV requires almost no calories so even if we are awake that does not justify needing to eat those extra calories. The result is fat gained and the creation of the late night myth! If clients find themselves struggling to not eat late, I always recommend creating a routine that gets them to bed and sleeping at an hour that does not leave them tired and eating to maintain alertness. Does all that make sense?"

"I think so; but I have another question now. I have also heard that I should not weight myself very often but that I should weigh my food, is that true?"

"No and Yes. When I first started helping people with fat loss I had been instructed by the then current experts to not have clients weigh more frequently than once every ten days or so. Since then there has been research showing that people who weigh more frequently lose more fat quicker and keep it off longer! So, I suggest weighing yourself as often as is mentally healthy for you."

"What do you mean by that?"

"I mean that you should do it as often as you can without it making you feel defeated or so obsessed with it that you cannot fully function in other areas of your life. You want a healthy, attractive body and that means having a healthy lifestyle too. The way to a healthy lifestyle is balance between your mind, body, and spirit. If you are neglecting other things in your life, such as relationships with other people, you will not succeed in your quest for health and happiness!"

The man indicated that he understood so the trainer continued, "The yes to your original question about weighing food is that there is overwhelming evidence that people who weigh and measure their food are *far* more likely to reach their goals. A big part of this is having focus on your habits and a bigger part of this is that when a person guesses about the quantity of food and the calories in it he underestimates the amount by up to **50%**![8] Studies have shown that lean people underestimate their foods' calories by 20% and overweight people underestimate by30-50%! He thinks he is doing good but is not. A compounding factor to this is that when we have food available we eat it, even though we are just as satisfied with a smaller portion.[9]

Closely related to weighing and measuring is logging food. Recent research was conducted with people tracking their calorie intake. They discovered that people who log their food intake at least 5 days per week had the best results. Those people lost twice the

---

[8] www.dotfit.com/content-1453.html

[9] Rolls BJ, Morris EL, Roe LS. Portion size of food affects energy intake in normal-weight and overweight men and women. *American Journal of Clinical Nutrition.* 2002; 76:1207-1213.

weight as people who do not and they kept it off longer! A different study found that people who tracked their food in a log over the holidays actually lost weight and they were not even on a nutrition plan or diet! It was the mere fact of paying attention to consumption that changed their behavior![10] They *knew* what they were putting into their mouths!" He paused for effect. "How much space does one cup of juice take up?"

The man indicated with his hands, "About a glass full."

"That is exactly what most people think but it is closer to a little less than half a typical glass! So, had you consumed your guess then you would have overeaten!"

"I see." He said as the trainer handed him another card. This one read:

> # IF YOU GUESS, YOUR RESULTS WILL
> # REFLECT IT!

"Is that why it is so easy for us to get fat? We are always guessing and so we guess wrong and get more and more fat?"

"Yes. But there is more to it than that. There are two main reasons that we have gotten fatter as a society. There is a kind of conspiratorial drama that plays out in our bodies around 30—give or take a couple years. To fully appreciate this conspiracy you need to understand the concept of homeostasis."

"Oh, I am sure I'll regret this but what is that?" He asked smiling.

He gave the man a feigned look of indignity, "You asked for it! The concept of homeostasis is that your body wants to maintain where it is in all functions; and it wants to

---

[10] Baker, RC, Kirshenbaum DS. Weight control during the holidays: Highly consistent self-monitoring as a potentially useful coping mechanism. *Health Psychology.* 1998; 17:367-370.

do this as efficiently as possible! This function is what allows people in impoverished areas of the world to survive. It is built into our genetic code to be efficient in all physiologic processes and to minimize energy expenditure. This really works against us in the U.S. in two ways. First, it works against us in that we always want to eat so that we have a store of energy, our fat, for a proverbial rainy day when a person does not have enough food intake for the expenditures his body makes. This is great in developing countries and in the past where and when people did not have access to food. But we are in the extraordinarily unique position where we always have food available and have not had those 'rainy days'. So, our bodies keep storing and storing the energy. Secondly, and more directly related to the point is that to be efficient with energy our bodies constantly monitor use of materials and their relative worth."

"I have no idea what you are saying."

"Okay…" He paused to reformulate his answer before continuing. " Our body is made of many different tissue types that require different levels of energy to maintain. A pound of fat only requires 4 calories per day to maintain. You need a blood supply to it, to keep it at body temperature, and that is almost it. Other materials that are not fat require more energy, some up to 55 calories per day per pound![11] So, if your body does not *need* to have that tissue then it gets rid of it. The problem with that is you end up burning less calories in a day, we call it…"

"A slow metabolism!" The man interjected.

---

[11] Elia, M. Organ tissue contribution to metabolic rate. In: Energy Metabolism: Tissue Determinants and Cellular Corollaries, edited by J.M. Kinney. New York: Raven © 1992, p. 61-77.

"Right!" He said excitedly. "We decrease our metabolism in part by losing tissue that requires a lot of energy to maintain. Research in the U.S. and Western Europe has shown that the average person loses about a pound of fat free mass each year and gains a little less than one pound of fat mass every year from the age of 25 on. Our bodies get rid of those tissues that require high amounts of energy to maintain but are not used. Eventually you figure that the monthly cost is not worth it and you cancel it. This physiological phenomenon happens in places around the world where we have removed physical labor and recreation from life. We used to think that muscle, strength, and bone loss was a natural process of aging. After this research it was discovered that these decrements of aging were the result of lifestyles without the stimulation to *need* fat free mass not from aging alone.[12] People who stimulated their bodies to *need* fat free mass do not lose it at the same rate as those people who are sedentary. Thinking about it in financial terms again, we could say that your body does not want to spend energy on things it does not need for survival or use often. It is like cancelling the gym membership that costs you $30 per month but you never use it. That means that if the fat free mass is on the high end of the caloric requirement (55 calories) then there will be a 51 calorie surplus everyday if the person does not change anything else in her life. After 5 years the person will have a 251-calorie surplus everyday! Seven days per week and 52 weeks a year! Compounding all this is the fact that around 30 your body completes its final major building project—fusion of your spine at the sacrum, or back of your pelvis. Well, around that 30 mark we have had 5ish years of fat free mass loss, our spine stops growing, and we typically begin focusing on careers and kids. We spend less time being active and do not have much weight-bearing on the bones and muscles to require them to be maintained."

---

[12] Wilmore JH, Costill DL, Kenney WL. (2008) *Physiology of sport and exercise.* 4th ed. Champaign, IL: Human Kinetics. p. 406

"Sounds like a losing battle."

"Yes, but only if you don't know about it and let it happen. When we don't know about it, out of habit, we continue to eat the same as we used to but do not need anywhere close to the same amount of caloric intake. That is why people begin noticing a huge weight gain around that time in their lives. They do not understand calories-in versus calories-out and that they now have far fewer calories going out! The fact is, based off the laws of physics, there can be no weight gain without excess calories. When someone tells me that they have been eating 'good' and within their calorie range but still gain fat I have no choice but to call them for what they are—'a cheater, cheater closet eater.' They are not admitting (even to themselves) how much they are consuming."

"I see why people say that nutrition is 80% of my success!"

The trainer held up his hand, "Hold on there; nutrition is extremely important but that is overstating it! Nutrition will make or break a person's attempt to change her body but other factors are vitally important too. You cannot get the healthy, attractive body you want without the other Factors too! You need to have a good supplement regimen, a resistance and cardio program, and a support structure. Without any of these Factors you will never be the fit, healthy person who you want to become."

"Because those other Factors are the other half of the equation—the expenditure side?" The man asked.

The trainer shook his head affirmatively. "That and the fact that motivation and routine redesign is essential for long-term success. Remember that knowing and doing are two very different things! I have tried to simplify it for you, but simple and easy are two very different things. Knowing that you should not eat at a fast-food place is common sense, but not easy;

especially after a hard day of work and having a couple kids to feed! It's simple to say 'Don't eat there', but it is not always easy when you have fussy kids in the back seat and are exhausted!

I think that we have covered enough for the day. You have been given a lot of new information to process! Remember that calories in versus calories out is the key to your fat loss success!" He handed the man another card.

FACTOR ONE

Nutrition:

- Calories-in vs. Calories-out

- Balance Your Macronutrients

- Manage Your Hormones

- Congratulations! You have mastered the First Factor!

"Of course you have not really passed the First Factor yet. You don't do that until you have demonstrated the ability to *apply* those points and that knowledge to your lifestyle! There will be a test on this—and the grade is determined by how you live and how your body changes!"

"I get it."

"I believe that you do! Let's stop here for now, put into practice what we've discussed and next week we will take on Factor 2!"

The man collected his cards, packed his bag, and took his leave. Once again he was tired but excited. He had learned so many things today that his head was nearly spinning and he knew that his time, energy, and money had been well spent. For the first time in his life he felt that he might have an understanding of how the whole food thing works with fitness and how he might be able to make changes! His excitement overrode his fatigue and he nearly jogged out of the building.

The next week he came back with a little less pep in his step and a look of concern on his face. He was hesitant to look the trainer in the eyes when he approached the desk.

"Things did not go as well as you hoped?" The trainer asked as he drew near.

"No." He said, his being permeating shame.

The trainer stood up and put a hand on his shoulder. "It's okay. We all have our own journey to make with health and fitness, especially regarding food. It is okay to make mistakes as long as we learn from them and do better next time. You will do better next time, right?"

"Yes... It was the darn eating out that got me. I could not figure out the calories and it was hard to stop eating before I had finished it all." His eyes were still looking at the floor.

"It is really hard to eat out and be successful with weight loss."

"I guess that I need to stop eating out, huh?"

"Actually, no. You just need to plan it better. People who successfully lose weight dine out an average of 2.5 times per week, including one time at a fast food restaurant.[13] Surprising, isn't it?" He continued after the man shook his head and looked up. "What we need to do is cook on the weekends so that you have enough food to last the week and reduce your need to eat out. When you do eat out I want you to choose the foods on this list because they are high in fiber, which only partially digests and has half the calories of other foods."

"And it is all about calories-in and calories-out!" The man was starting to perk back up.

"Right, and vegetables are a great way to do it. They are high in fiber and you can add them to soups, sauté them to top rice, or eat them raw! I also want to create a food rewards calendar with you. We will pick three goals to work on this next week and three rewards you get when you accomplish those goals."

The trainer pulled out his measuring tools and took he man's body composition, circumference measurements, and weight. He worked out the numbers and revealed to the man that his disappointment was justified—he had not lost any weight and even gained a little fat! This was not how it was supposed to go!

They worked for quite a while and after a bit of back and forth they finally forged a plan that they agreed was both workable and productive! He would only eat out three times that next week, include fresh vegetables in two snacks per day, and reduce his soft drink consumption to four cans during the week. As a reward for accomplishing two of these three goals he decided he would treat himself to a new movie at the theater! Once again the man left with improved spirits and a renewed optimism.

---

[13] Wing, RR. Hill JO. *Annual Review of Nutrition.* 2001; 21:323-341.

The week passed quickly and he struggled through parts of it and had to focus on what the trainer had told him. He began to truly understand what the trainer meant by the statement that simple and easy were not the same thing! Through grit and determination he willed himself to success; fighting through the temptations and routines he emerged on the other end of the week victorious over his hunger, bad habits, and nutrition—he felt great both physically and mentally! The weight of food-bondage and past failures felt lighter and he basked in the feeling of measured control that he had never known before. He had begun to free himself from the mind-forged manacles that had enslaved him for so long—freedom had never felt so good! He knew that he had not learned enough to get where he wanted to be or to make it last forever so it was with eager anticipation that he returned to the trainer for their next session. He could hardly wait to tell the trainer about his week and how he had mastered food!

Factor Two

Nutritional Supplementation

(or Cellular Triage)

When the man entered the room for his next appointment the trainer was seated behind the table again, only this time it was stacked with supplement bottles on the right side and had a platter with a hunk of raw bloody meat on the left.

"Before we begin on Factor Two tell me how your week went."

The man excitedly told of his success and how he had accomplished it. The trainer congratulated him with equal enthusiasm. They discussed why and where he succeeded as well as why and where he failed. Next they devised plans for the next week for overcoming the problems he had experienced. Once that was settled they turned back to the table and its contents.

"What's with the bloody meat?"

"That, my friend, is a liver! Looks tasty, right!" Said the trainer as he plunged a carving fork into it.

The man suppressed a shudder responding, "No thanks. I think that I will pass."

"You and me both! I thought you might say that, most people do. The reason that I put it out there is that there is only one study I have read where a person can eat all the nutrients they need to stay healthy; guess what was on the menu?"

"Umm...Liver?"

"Kinda obvious with the slab sitting there, huh? Yes, Registered Dietitians were tasked with designing menus that met the 1989 RDAs and the 1990 Dietary Guidelines while keeping the calories between 2,200 and 2,400 and being palatable.[14][15] Most the menus did not meet all the nutritional requirements but the one that was able to find a way to get them all in did it through eating liver twice daily."

"Yuck!"

"I know, right! I don't want to eat it once, let alone twice a day everyday! The problem was compounded by the fact that it required an average female to be in a caloric surplus—causing them to gain fat! Part of the cause is the decreasing nutrient value in grocery foods. Because of antiquated farming techniques and land overuse our foods now have 15-20% fewer nutrients than 20 years ago.[16][17] Also, genetic engineering has changed food to look ripe before it is, last longer on the shelves, and resist insects. These changes nutritionally devalue the foods![18] The point is that it is not realistic to expect yourself to eat all the nutrients your body needs to both change and remain healthy. On top of all that is the fact that you need to create a caloric deficit in order to lose fat..."

---

[14] Dollahite J, Franklin D, McNew R. Problems encountered in meeting the Recommended Dietary Allowances for menus designed according to the Dietary Guidelines for Americans. *Journal of the American Dietitians Association.* 1995; 95:341-344, 347.

[15] Krebs-Smith SM, Guenther PM, Subar AF, Kirkpatrick SI, Dodd KW. Americans do not meet federal dietary recommendations. *Journal of Nutrition.* 2010 Oct;140(10):1832-8. Epub 2010 Aug 11.

[16] Comb GF. The vitamins, fundamental aspects in nutrition and health. Second Edition. San Diego: Academic Press; 1998. 469-79.

[17] Kant AK. Reported consumption of low-nutrient-density foods by American children and adolescents: nutritional and health correlates, NHANES III, 1988 to 1994. *Archives of Pediatric and Adolescent Medicine.* 2003 Aug;157(8):789-96.

[18] Shils ME, Vernon RY. Modern Nutrition in health and disease. 7th edition. Philadelphia PA: Lea and Febiger;1988. 1694.

"That Law of Physics!"

"Exactly! The First Law of Thermodynamics—if you want to lose fat you must be in a caloric deficit and that means not consuming enough calories for your body's output! If you cannot get enough nutrients with a normal caloric intake then there is no way to get them taking less than that!"

"So, how do I lose fat while staying healthy?"

"That is what we use multivitamins for! They are nutrients without calories! Back in 2002 the U.S. Surgeon General announced that all U.S. citizens should take a multivitamin because 70% of ALL our health problems are nutritionally related. In fact, the World Health Organization estimated that 97% of Americans have some sort of nutritional deficiency and the Journal of the American Medical Association recommended "that ALL adults take a multi-vitamin daily."[19] Many other organizations then jumped on the bandwagon after that.[20] It may seem like this is common sense but it was not too long ago when the entire supplement industry was looked down upon and doctors often did not recommend the use of supplements."

"Why was that?"

"Because the industry is not regulated by the Food and Drug Administration (FDA). Back in 1996 Congress passed the DSHEA ACT, which effectively kicked out the Feds from regulating supplements![21] The result has been a slough of poorly made products that don't do what they claim, don't have the advertised ingredients, or have weak potency! The industry is about making money and since they are able to cut corners without repercussion; they do!"

---

[19] *The Journal of the American Medical Association.* June 19, 2002
[20] Marra MV, Boyar AP. Position of the American Dietetic Association: nutrient supplementation. *Journal of American Dietitians Association.* 2009 Dec;109(12):2073-85.
[21] www.fda.gov/food/DietarySupplements/default.htm. Retrieved 12/09/2012.

"So why would I want to take any?"

"Because there are a handful of companies that pay extra to pharmaceutical manufactures so they can insure the quality of their products. They have products that are made of pure and potent ingredients with delivery systems that work, making them both safe and effective. The only way to insure you are taking these products is to use products made in a fully licensed, federally registered manufacturing facility. These facilities and are regularly inspected by the FDA because they are required to follow very strict quality guidelines and Good Manufacturing Practices (GMPs).[22] GMPs are extremely important procedures that insure quality manufacturing. Good companies subject themselves to the GMP procedure and additional testing to make certain that a product has optimum bioavailability and digestibility!"

"Bio—what?" the man stopped him.

"Bioavailability. It means that not only is a nutrient present in a supplement but it also is in a form that the body can absorb during digestion."

"If it is digested why wouldn't it get absorbed?"

"Now your thinking! Good!" He said with a gleam in his eye. He loved to see people learning to master the Five Factors of Fitness! "The answer is counterintuitive—no. Just because it is broken down does not mean your body will absorb it; sometimes they just pass through! The main reason that this happens is that the micronutrients are not properly enrobed." Seeing his forehead crinkle quizzically the trainer quickly answered the question he knew was coming. "Enrobement can be thought of as a protective suit around each vitamin and mineral. The enzymes and acid of the digestive tract from the mouth through the small intestine are constantly bombarding these suits to crack them open and get the nutrients. The problem is that only certain areas within the digestive tract can actually absorb certain micronutrients. For example, the first part of the small intestine, the Duodenum,

---

[22]www.fda.gov/food/DietarySupplements/GuidanceComplianceRegulatoryInformation/RegulationsLaws/ucm173996.htm. Retrieved 12/09/2012.

absorbs Calcium but the latter parts of the small intestine, the Jejunum and Ileum, cannot
absorb it. Similarly, the Jejunum is where Vitamin C is absorbed and the Ileum is where
Vitamin A is absorbed.[23] If the suit is cracked too soon the nutrient is destroyed before it can
make it to where it is absorbed. Similarly if it is cracked too late it cannot be absorbed further
down the tract. It must be released at precisely the right moment, or place, to be absorbed."

"Wow! I had no idea it was so complicated!"

"Most people don't, which is why companies can cut corners and produce inferior
products."

"Can't I just take a bunch of something and know that at least some of it will get through
to be absorbed?"

"You could; but everything we consume has a level, that if passed, makes it toxic to our
systems. Through experimentation, scientists have determined the level of exposure to each
micronutrient at which significant problems are first observed; it is called the Lowest
Observed Adverse Effect Level."[24]

"Too much of a good thing is a bad thing?"

"Exactly! I am going to have to steal that from you and make it into one of my cards!"

"The man grinned, "Thanks; feel free to. I am just glad I am getting this stuff!"

"So yes, too much is bad and so we need to put in the right amount to stay healthy. When
we eat food and our bodies work properly our systems are designed to help tell us what to eat
and when to stop. I won't beat that dead horse about satiety we talked about during Factor
One but here is a place it comes into play; if we don't eat right then our bodies don't work
properly. Since our bodies are not working properly and we need an artificial means of
nutrient delivery the supplements have to be precise!"

---

[23] www.siumed.edu/mic/research/nutrient/gi42sg.html

[24] www.epa.gov/risk_assessment/glossary.htm

"If they are not regulated, how precise are the popular ones? It seems that they would not be all that good." The man interjected.

He nodded, "Right you are! When I first began helping people with fat loss I watched one of those exposé shows like 20/20 or Dateline where they did a series of tests on the most popular multivitamins and found that they only had an nutrient uptake of around 10% of the advertised nutrients."

"Really? That's pathetic!"

"I know—right! The only thing that the FDA checked them for was that they dissolved in an acid the same pH as our stomach acid. So, all these brands cut corners and produced poor products. The good news is that they did dissolve and people did not have a bunch of pills filling their stomachs! These days many companies are producing products using GMPs but few subject themselves to the additional testing to insure delivery systems for bioavailability."

"That's all fascinating, but what does it have to do with me?" Puzzled the man.

"We need you to get the nutrients into your body so that you can be healthy while you lose the fat. When your body is deprived of the micronutrients it needs, it has to perform a kind of 'cellular triage'."[25]

"Triage? I thought that was something they do in hospital ERs?"

He indicated 'sort of' with his head and hands, "Well, triage is a French term that originates from battlefield medicine.[26] It is a system to categorize and place people into defined groups based on the surgeons' estimate of most likely to survive. They would put people who were hopelessly injured in one area and not waste time treating them—they were

---

[25] Ames BN. Low micronutrient intake may accelerate the degenerative diseases of aging through allocation of scarce micronutrients by triage. Proc Natl Acad Sci U S A. 2006 Nov 21;103(47):17589-94. Epub 2006 Nov 13. Review.

[26] www.medical-dictionary.thefreedictionary.com/triage

expected to only get worse regardless of any medical assistance. The next group was anyone who was severely injured, had a chance to survive with help, but did not require immediate attention. The final group was comprised of people who were injured in a way that if they had immediate attention they would survive—these people were treated first because they needed it first! They had to do this because the number of wounded soldiers so vastly outnumbered the supply of surgeons and tools! In this way they saved the most lives possible given the circumstances!"

"I think that's a sad story! But I get the connection. My body has a limited supply of nutrients and has to make decisions about where to send them. The most vital and important functions are satisfied first and then it goes down the line of importance until it is out of supply. Those functions that do not get the nutrients often contribute to what you told me earlier about the disease process. The diseases are able to take hold and corrupt those cells." The man paused and asked, "But what I do not understand is why doesn't everyone losing weight get sick or a disease?"

"Impressive! You made the perfect connection! Before I tell you the answer to your very perceptive question, take this card." He said handing him another card that had written on it:

Cellular Triage:

- Your body uses nutrients for optimal health.

- Lacking nutrients makes you SICK!

- Being SICK makes changing harder and less fun!

After he took the card, the trainer told him, "To answer your question, it is because when a person is in a caloric deficit (but not getting the proper nutrients) they do not always get sick right away. What happens is that the body begins to cannibalize its fat free mass, because it is so calorically expensive. For these people each pound of weight lost is a fourth fat free mass and *three*-fourths fat mass![27] This ends with the same results as the 30 year-old scenario—people burn far less than they had before and it catches up to them!"

"And that is why I need supplements!"

"Right, back to the idea of the FDA and regulations! Don't you think that quality, purity and results are what is most important when it comes to your health? Rather than the Wednesday "buy-one, get one free" special, or your neighbor's multi-level marketing of the month sales pitch? Buying products from non-GMP sources to save a few dollars will ultimately cost you in the long run. You will not get your results, your health will suffer, and you will have wasted money!"

"I see now. That makes sense. If I can't eat the things that make me healthy because of their calories I need to take them in with supplements that have no calories. These need to come from a manufacturer who pays extra to be regulated for the important aspects of supplements—purity, potency, and delivery!" The man stated while reflecting on his time wasted with T.V. products; no wonder they never worked!

---

[27] http://www.dotfit.com/content-5435.html?utm_source=iContact&utm_medium=email&utm_campaign=B2B%20Prospects&utm_content=, Retrieved 12/09/2012.

The trainer nodded. "You do get it!" He pulled a card out of his desk and handed it to him. It read:

FACTOR TWO

Supplements:

Good Manufacturing Practices Guarantee:

1. Purity

2. Potency

3. Delivery Systems

The man snatched up the card, "Does this mean I passed the Second Factor?"

The trainer held up his hand, "Whoa! Hold your horses. We have just scratched the surface! This was just the foundation for this Factor of Fitness; now we need to discuss the specifics of Meal Replacements, Lipotropics, and Thermogenics. Your multivitamin combined with these three supplements will be the four pillars of your supplement regimen."

"I knew that had to be too easy."

The trainer stood up and placed the liver in a cooler next to the table before continuing, "Why do you think that eating right is so hard?"

After pondering the question for a moment the man said, "I think that it is just so difficult to eat those types of food that people can't do it."

The trainer nodded, "You're correct! The challenge of healthy eating is convenience and quality! When you say it is so 'different' you mean that it is not our typical manner of eating; it takes preparation and time, which people feel is inconvenient! Also, acquiring the right quality, you called 'types', can take time and effort. All this is much more demanding than going to a restaurant, cooking a frozen dinner, or grabbing takeout! We can address these issues by using supplements named 'Meal Replacements'. Meal replacements have been shown to help people lose fat two times quicker and keep it off longer!"[28]

"That's not too surprising. I have always felt better after eating a PowerBar!"

"You have to be careful which type of bar you consume and make certain that it is a *meal* replacement, not a Protein *Supplement*."

"What's the difference?"

"A Protein supplement is designed to increase your intake of protein and a meal replacement is designed to increase your intake of carbohydrates, proteins, and fats. The best ones have the ratio of 60% carbohydrates, 20% proteins, and 20% fats; sound familiar?"

"Um…vaguely?" The man said shrugging his shoulders.

"Remember in Factor One about the typical ratio of macronutrients for people to be healthy, satisfied, and energetic being 60/20/20?"

"Oh, yes! That's why!"

"Right. You give a person correct quality macronutrients in a convenient form and simple is made easy! When people seeking to lose fat use meal replacement they have the convenience and quality wrapped into one, making proper eating easier!"

---

[28] Heynsfield SB, van Mierlo CA, van der Knaap HC, Heo M, Frier HI. Weight management using a meal replacement strategy. Meta and pooling analysis from six studies. *International Journal of Obesity Related Disorders.* (2003) May, 27 (5): 537-49.

"So if I get what you are saying, when I use a meal replacement I will have the quick, convenient food I want but it also keeps my calories under control as well as keeping me satisfied and healthy!" He said with a smile.

The trainer nodded his head, "Exactly! You really are beginning to master these concepts—great work! Now let's talk about the next type of supplement you will need to be successful. This group is called 'Lipotropics' and they are essential for your health and your goal of fat loss. Do you remember what I measured your body fat percentage at during our first meeting?"

He shook his head 'no', "I only remember that I was in an unhealthy category and that I was at risk for some health problems."

The trainer pulled out a client file from the desk and opened it, "Correct, you were measured at 25%, which is in the category of 'unhealthy'. When a person is in that category they develop a condition called Fatty Liver Syndrome.[29] This is a condition where the liver is not metabolizing fat at the rate that it should be. Think of the liver as a sink drain and the water as fat storage. When the liver functions correctly it 'drains' the fat at a normal rate but if the liver is 'fatty' it is like a clogged sink drain. The fat drains slowly and it takes longer to empty the sink. This makes it hard to lose fat and your body may cannibalize more easily accessed fat free mass to meet the energy needs."[30]

"Which is bad because fat free mass is your body's best fat-burning machinery!"

---

[29] Jiang J, Torok N. Nonalcoholic steatohepatitis and the metabolic syndrome. *Metabolic Syndrome Related Disorders.* 2008 Spring;6(1):1-7. Review.
[30] Dulloo AG, Antic V, Montani JP. Ectopic fat stores: housekeepers that can overspill into weapons of lean body mass destruction. *International Journal of Obesity Related Metabolic Disorders.* 2004 Dec;28 Suppl 4:S1-2.

"Right! What a lipotropic supplement does is restore your liver closer to its naturally functioning level of fat metabolism, prevents dietary fat storage, and increases fat loss by up to 2-3 times![31] The active ingredients in these are a combination of herbs and amino acids. Does that all make sense?"

"Yes. It helps my sink drain normally!" He smiled.

He returned the smile, "If by 'sink' you mean 'liver' and if by 'drain' you mean 'metabolize fat' then you are correct! The next supplement group is called thermogenics."

"I remember those; I have taken some of them. The salesman told me that they helped burn calories by wasting energy in your body even when I was not working out. I don't think that they worked; I never lost weight and I never even felt warmer." The man stated.

"Even when a thermogenic supplement is properly made you will not feel warmer; the increase in calorie usage is on such a small scale, 3-5%, it is not noticeable.[32] But you are correct that the extra calorie use is happening outside of workouts. It works by using pyruvate, something found naturally in food like apples, to trigger extra metabolic cycles of cellular energy production, which requires calories to do."

The man stopped him with a raised hand, "Why not just eat the apples?"

"That would make sense except that you would need to eat a barrel of apples to get the level of necessary levels of pyruvate!"

"No thanks. And it would violate the calories in versus calories out principle!" He said looking pleased with himself.

---

[31] Abidov T, Grachev SV, Klimenov AL, Kalynzhih OV. Effects of Rhododendron caucasicum extract on body weight and dietary lipid absorption in obese patients: A double-blind placebo controlled clinical study. Final Report: Russian Ministry of Health; Grant: No: 03-122-1997; Clinical Study Study; Project No: 0101-1997/ 8pp.
[32] www.dotfit.com/content-3657.html

"Right again; you really did your homework this week! It becomes counterproductive to try and eat your way to the results. Remember supplementation is all about nutrients *without* the calories!" He said as he handed him another card:

Supplementation: Nutrients without calories!

"There is one more supplement that we are going to take while you are trying to lose fat—fish oil. Fish oil has been found to help people lose fat and slightly increase fat free mass!"[33]

"Can't I just eat fish in my meals? You have said that eating food closest to its natural state is the best to do." He inquired.

"Typically that is the case but research in this specific area has shown that using a supplement gives more fat loss with greater reduction in waist circumference than eating actual fish."[34]

" A smaller waist? I'm sold!" He exclaimed.

They went online to DotFit, a research and development company who practices GMPs with their products, and ordered the supplements that they had discussed. The man was given instructions on when to expect them shipped to his home and how to take them properly.

---

[33] Hill AM, Buckley JD, Murphy KJ, Howe PR: Combining fish-oil supplements with regular aerobic exercise improves body composition and cardiovascular disease risk factors. *American Journal of Clinical Nutrition* 2007, 85:1267-1274.

[34] Thorsdottir I, Tomasson H, Gunnarsdottir I, Gisladottir E, Kiely M, Parra MD, Bandarra NM, Schaafsma G, Martinez JA: Randomized trial of weight-loss-diets for young adults varying in fish and fish oil content. *International Journal of Obesity* (Lond) 2007, 31:1560-1566.

They set an appointment for a week later and the man went home to process all the new information that he had received.

The week went by quickly and the man had a hectic week at work. He knew that he had eaten poorly and that he had missed a few of his supplements throughout the week. When he came to the next appointment he was prepared for not having made much progress but was flabbergasted to be measured with an *increase* in his fat percentage! He could hardly believe it! This could not be happening again!

"I can hardly believe this!" He exclaimed.

Seeing his frustration the trainer realized that the man needed a morale boost. "How many times did you eat out this past week?" He inquired.

"Only once! It's not fair!" He said flushed with irritation.

"Fairness has nothing to do with it. Remember, it is governed by laws of physics—you get what you put into it! However, you are making progress; keep that in mind! Before we started meeting you ate out how many times per week?"

"Every day, sometimes twice a day."

"Right, now you are down to once per week! And you said that you are sleeping better and more energetic, right!"

"Yes. That's true!"

"So, don't get down on yourself! This is a journey; if it was easy everyone would be in good shape—but they are not! Celebrate your successes! Keep your chin up and keep attacking it and it will eventually all come together! Now let's tackle the challenges you had with supplementation."

"I had trouble remembering to take a meal replacement to work for my morning snack so there were a few days when I went out to the coffee shop and grabbed a bagel or muffin; but I forgot to ask for a nutrition sheet. I guess my results reflect my guessing, huh."

"Yes. But remember how far you have come. Now you know *why* you are not doing good and *how* you could have done better! Those are huge steps in the right direction! This week I want you to put your meal replacements in your lunch bag the night before work. This way you will be less likely to forget it, okay?" He said enthusiastically and handed him another card.

FACTOR TWO

Nutritional Supplementation:

- Cellular Triage

- Good Manufacturing Practices

- Nutrients without Calories

- Congratulations! You have mastered the Second Factor!

The man collected his cards, set their next appointment and went home. He did what the trainer had suggested and found that the Second Factor was easier to master than the First, with which he still was struggling.

Factor Three

Cardiovascular Training

(or Heart Healthy Calorie Burn)

The next time the man entered the room for his appointment the trainer was waiting with a stopwatch, towel, and water bottle. "Today we are going to the gym for cardio! You got my message about wearing workout clothes I see!" He said indicating the outfit the man was wearing.

"Yep." He replied following him down the hallway.

They went through a rigorous cardio workout and the trainer met him in the office after he showered. He walked into the room ruddy-faced and his body and mind fully awakened. "That was great! I feel so...so..."

"Alive?" He asked.

"Yes! Alive! Like I'm a superhero in a sci-fi movie who senses everything! Is that normal?"

"Yes; in the beginning at least. It is a phenomenon called EPOC. That is an acronym for Exercise Post Oxygen Consumption. It is a term for the metabolic processes that occur immediately following an intense exercise session. Remember what we had discussed about efficiency and the body making changes to be the most effective it can be? Well, this is another perfect example of that. When a person's body is not accustomed to a certain stress it will spend energy to improve itself to be better capable of handling that stress the next time it occurs. During that time the body is on high alert, fully engaged and hot because of the energy being used to repair and modify cellular structures. You look hot right now, are you?"

The man dabbed his forehead with his hand towel, "Yes. I am starting to sweat again!"

"That's EPOC! You are sweating because of the energy your body is using to change for the better!"

"I have worked out often in the past and didn't always get this feeling, why is that?"

"Excellent question! There is only so much change your body can undergo before it is at peak proficiency at a task. Once that level of proficiency is reached, the body no longer can make adjustments for improvements."

"It's as good as it can get?! Is this the dreaded 'plateau' that everyone tries to avoid?"

"Yes it is. It is important to understand that EPOC basically is a two-for-one event. You burn calories to perform the exercise and then you burn calories after the exercise when your body is rebuilding and improving itself! I don't know about you but I want to get the most out of my time; if I can get 30 minutes of cardio benefit with 20 minutes of work that is what I want to do! When the plateau happens the person still gets the benefits of the 20 minutes of cardio but not the extra '10 minutes' of energy burn. Luckily there is a way to avoid the loss of EPOC. We call it the FITT principle."

"Let me guess, another acronym?"

"Right. This one stands for Frequency, Intensity, Time, and Type. If you change any of these correctly you can maintain EPOC because your body is always having to adjust to the different stimuli." He said handing him a card:

F.I.T.T. Principle:

Frequency

Intensity

Time

Type

Taking the card he said, "I think I get it. Frequency is how many days per week I do it, Intensity I am not sure what you mean by that, Time is how long I do it for, and Type is what I am doing for my cardio."

"That's correct! You nailed Frequency, Time, and Type so let me explain Intensity. Intensity is the level of difficulty you perform your cardio at. There are two common ways that we judge this. The first is with a person's heart rate. We often hear and read about Target Heart Rates and this is what they are referring to—the intensity of an exercise. There are many misleading ideas with the concept of Target Heart Rate. The most common is that a lower heart rate will burn more fat and that fat loss exercisers should work out at that lower level. This is another half-truth! There is more energy used from body fat during exercise in that range but fat loss is about the total energy deficit at the end of the day. It does not matter if the energy came from fat, glucose, or glycogen the only thing that matters is that there is an energy deficit! If you burn more calories in a higher intensity workout you will lose more fat! The second common way people judge the intensity of a workout is called the Perceived Rate of Exertion. This is a scale of how hard you are working in relation to your prior experiences; a one is very light and a ten is very, very heavy. The ideal on this method is to be out of breath enough to talk but not carry on a conversation, usually at a 3 or 4 on the scale.

Did you take your resting heart rate like I asked?"

He nodded his head. "Yes. I did it just like you asked: right after I woke up and before getting out of bed. It was 64 beats per minute."

"Using what is called the Karvonen formula we can calculate your target heart rate. The formula is **{[(220-Age) − resting HR] × %Intensity} + resting HR=Target Heart Rate.** You told me that you have recently turned 32, so let's plug that into the formula and figure out what your rate would be for an intensity of 65%. So, you take 220-32, which equals 188. Then we take the 188 from your resting heart rate of 64, which equals 124. After that we multiply the 124 with .65, which is the percent intensity at which I want you to start."

He stopped the trainer with an upraised hand, "How did you get .65 from 65%?"

"To make a decimal from a percentage you take the 65% and move the decimal over to the right two places."

"Oh yeah! I remember that from math class! So, if I wanted to work out a higher intensity I could do a .75 or if I wanted a lower intensity I could calculate it at a .55!"

"So you get it then? Good. At that point we take the 124 and multiply it by .65, which equals 80.6. After we get that number we add your resting heart rate of 64 back in to get the target heart rate of 144.6, which I would round to 145 beats per minute! That is the heart rate you need to be exercising at for an intensity of 65%!"

"And you showed me this because you want me to know how to adjust my target heart rate as my resting rate improves with my fitness and as I age, right?"

Exactly! Let's get back to EPOC, the important thing to remember about intensity is that it gets changed to keep your body having to burn calories to adjust."

"That almost makes it sound like you can make it harder or *easier*." He said.

"Actually, you are correct. To keep EPOC going moving your intensity up *or* down will have the same effect. The key is to change one of the other aspects to compensate for the loss of intensity if you decrease it."

"Are you saying that if I decrease my intensity I need to increase my time or frequency to make up the difference?"

"Yes. If you had been at a heart rate of 145 beats per minute and reduce it to 130 beats per minute then you will need to increase the time spent at your workout, moving it from 20 minutes to 30 minutes *or* you could keep your time the same and increase your frequency from 3 days per week to 4 days per week. Something needs to change to keep you body guessing and changing! Does that all make sense? " He stated as he passed over a card that read:

Cardiovascular Training:

EPOC

Exercise

Post

Oxygen

Consumption

2 for 1 Special!

He took the card and nodded his head 'Yes' and wiped more sweat from his face, "But I thought that certain types of cardio are better than others?"

"It depends upon what you mean by 'better'. If you mean better at a certain activity than the answer is absolutely; the body becomes its function! If you want to swim better you need to focus on swimming more, not running or biking. If you mean 'better' at burning fat then the answer is not really. They are all so close in calorie burn that managing your EPOC is more important. The most important thing for you to consider after EPOC is which type of cardio *you* like and will do! The more you like it the more likely you will be to do it as often and as intense as you should!"

"Okay, what about when I do my cardio? I have read in magazines that I need to do it early in the morning before breakfast."

"This is just like your previous question—do cardio when *you* are most likely to do it! Back in Grad School we did a lab in my Exercise Physiology course where we monitored and charted our heart rate and temperature each waking hour. This showed each of us when our body was the most and least active during the day. Ideally, you want to exercise during the time of day when your body is at its peak energy. For me it was late morning to early afternoon. For others in my group it was early in the morning or late evening, when I was at my lowest point. We were all different! The trick is to structure your routines in a way that you can make it to the gym when your body is at its highest state of arousal so you can get the biggest bang for your buck! If you are disciplined and can do cardio during your resistance training session that would be best. First do your resistance training then do your cardio. The reason for this order is that cardio requires a lower intensity over a longer duration than resistance training. With resistance training we want close to maximal output, but it lasts a very short time. If you do your cardio first then you have tapped into some of the immediately available energy stored and have used that up. The problem is that you will not have that stored energy for the resistance exercises, which is really where it is needed. If you perform your resistance training first, you use the immediately available energy stores where they are needed and then still can perform your cardio at its best the level of intensity!" He said pulling a card out and handing it to the man.

"Sorry to change the subject but I have a cardio related question off this topic..." He timidly interrupted him, taking the card.

"Go ahead. The best learning comes from you and your thought processes!"

"You mentioned that it would be best if I did my cardio after my resistance workout, right?" He waited for an affirmative head nod, "Well, I was planning on doing some of those videos that incorporate weights into the workout to combine cardio with a weight lifting program. I don't want to get freaky huge like some of those bodybuilders."

"Unfortunately we will still need to do a resistance workout. Research has shown that traditional cardio does not pass the threshold that stimulates the maintenance or growth of fat free mass. In one study the researchers took cross sectional computed tomography (CTG) scans of three subjects' upper arms and performed a composition analysis on them.[35] The subjects were all 57-year-old males with similar body weights. One subject was sedentary, one was swimmer, and one was a resistance exerciser. Relative to the other two men, the sedentary man's arm bone had a larger center medullary cavity, which is that central hole where marrow is held, indicating a loss of bone density. His arm also had more subcutaneous body fat, which is the fat between the muscles and skin. He also had far less muscle tissue. The man who was swim trained had a medullary cavity slightly smaller than the first man, had larger triceps muscles, less subcutaneous body fat, and the same size of biceps muscles. The man who was strength trained had a far smaller medullary cavity and far larger biceps and triceps muscles. The study was one of many that showed that muscle and bone loss will occur when and where the body does not have enough stimuli to require that level of muscle or bone. The swimmer had enough to keep decent sized triceps but not biceps because of the type of resistance during the activity of swimming. All cardio activities are this way!"

"What about those classes I've seen that use hand weights in them?"

"Well, those still do not offer level of resistance needed to maintain or grow well-rounded fat-free mass. Remember the nature of a cardio activity is low intensity over a long

---

[35] Wilmore JH, Costill DL, Kenney WL. (2008) *Physiology of sport and exercise.* 4th ed. Champaign, IL: Human Kinetics. p. 408.

duration. This means the weights need to be light enough to be lifted so many times that they are not able to stimulate the growth of fat free mass; they become so light that they do not pass that threshold! This is exactly what we saw with the aforementioned study; the swimmer's biceps had resistance but not enough to keep their mass and size! We will discuss resistance training in more depth during the next Factor, just be warned that you *will* be doing resistance training if you want the healthy, athletic body you are looking for!"

The trainer stood up and shaking the man's hand said, "You are doing great! I usually do not have clients who ask such critically thought out questions. I believe that you will master the Five Factors of Fitness relatively quickly and will become a lifetime enthusiast of health and fitness!" He took out a card and handed it to the man.

FACTOR THREE

Cardiovascular Training:

- The F.I.T.T. Principle

- Do cardio classes or exercise with a friend!

- E.P.O.C—2 for 1 Special

- Do what you like!

- Do it when you will do it!

- Congratulations! You have mastered the Third Factor!

The man smiled, collected his cards, and set his next appointment. This was hard work! But it was becoming simpler! The fog was beginning to lift in his mind and things seemed to be coming together in a way that he understood. He was making the connections that he had known must be there!

The next three weeks were much easier than the previous ones and he felt a surge of pride and control about the progress he had been making! This made the news from his trainer all the more disappointing when he had his measurements retaken. Although he had not gained any fat since the previous measurement, he had not lost any either!

"But I did so good this time! I did it and felt so much better I was sure that I had made progress this time! This is so frustrating! I know it is not easy but I can't believe that I have not been losing any fat! I know that I am having all these other benefits of exercise but I want to *lose fat*! That is what we have been meeting for! Maybe I just don't have the right genetics. Maybe I am destined to be fat! I think that I am wasting my time and need to just accept who I am!" He frustratingly spat out in a whirlwind of negativity and disappointment.

Understanding the cathartic nature of expressing one's emotions the trainer allowed him to vent his frustration. When he had slowed down, began breathing more normally, and reason returned to his countenance the trainer said, "Let me tell you a story; it is a true story that has an enormous implication for you. Prior to the European settlement of the Southwestern U.S. and Mexico there lived a group of American Indians named the Pima. These people were farmers and worked hard in an inhospitable land to live. They farmed the riparian areas of a desert, scratching out a living amongst the cacti, mesquite trees, snakes, and sand. When the U.S. and Mexican governments established national borders the Pima were divided. Half of them lived north of the border in the U.S. and the other half lived south of the border in Mexico. Those in Mexico continued with their traditional form of farming, using livestock to plow their fields. They also ate a more traditional diet and had restricted access to alcohol. This group of the Pima were healthy and fit like their ancestors. The Pima in the U.S. were able to access modern machines to perform their farming work and normal U.S. access (unlimited!) to food, drink, and alcohol. In 2006 a massive study was conducted to discover the incidence of obesity and type 2 diabetes within these two groups. [36] The Pima in the south had incidences in line with the general Mexican population, which is far lower than the U.S. population. However, the Pima in the north, with all the trappings of our culture, had incidences far higher than their genetically identical counterparts in the south."

"So you are saying that the bottom line is that I could have genetics predisposed to obesity but that they are not the cause of the problem; it's that darn physics thing." He said, now much calmer.

"Yes. The Pima Indian Study and a plethora of twin studies have shown that genetics only play a small role in body fat."

"So they do play *a* role? How much and how can you be so sure that that is not what is happening to me?" The man inquired.

"Another good critical question! Because the studies show at most a 25% relation between genetics and obesity. The kicker is that the relationship is one of probability, not determination! That means that it increases a person's *chance* of gaining fat but not that they *will*. There is always choice involved and there still is no way to skirt around the First Law of Thermodynamics! Regardless of genetics you do not see pictures of obese concentration camp prisoners or anorexics because they do not consume enough energy to have extra stored

---

[36] Shultz LO, et al. (2006). Effects of traditional and western environments on prevalence of type 2 diabetes in Pima Indians in Mexico and the U.S., *Diabetes Care.* 29: 1866-1871.

as fat! Genetic predispositions only can express themselves given the right situations. For fat

storage, that means calories beyond the needs of the physiological functions and activities

performed! So, even *if* you had a strong predisposition to store fat you could not do it without

extra calories. We often do not want to own up to our shortcomings in life and this is an area

where people are notorious for not accepting responsibility for their actions; they want to

place the locus of control outside of their volition when it is anything but that!

I know of only one exception to volitional control as it relates to hunger and fat loss. It is

a genetic disorder called Prader-Willi Syndrome.[37] This is a genetic disorder that causes

intellectual disabilities, low muscle tone, decreased metabolism, and an inability to feel

satiated! These people, who luckily are only 1 in 15,000 births, do not have any of the normal

mechanisms to feel full! They always feel hungry, on the verge of starving hungry! You

would know if you had this though because of the symptoms that accompany it. These

symptoms require early interventions from therapists to move the child towards a more

normal life and almost always the disorder is 'caught' early in life."

"All that to say I have no real excuse?" The man joked.

"Correct! That and to encourage you towards success; when a person knows that his

actions determine what he becomes then he is more likely to do the right things. That is the

place I am attempting to lead you to!" He said pulling from his desk another card that read:

---

[37] http://fpwr.org/about-prader-willi-syndrome

<u>GENETICS AND FAT LOSS:</u>

- Genetics only predispose you!

- Lifestyle trumps genetics!

- Our decisions, not genetics, dictate our body!

The man took the card, placed it with his others, and left with a renewed optimism, if others can do it, then he can do it!! His genetics could not stop him, only his actions or inactions could! What a refreshing perspective! What an empowering perspective! He was the master of his body's destiny and it felt great!

That week passed quickly and all he had learned seemed to click. His body was responding to all the positive changes he had made! When he met with his trainer he had good news—he had lost 2 pounds of fat! The trainer congratulated him and explained that he could expect that rate of loss each week and possibly more once they implemented the final two Factors! It wasn't the crazy too-good-to-be-true 10 pounds in a week promises he had been given with diet books, special supplements, or TV gadgets—but those never felt this good and didn't have lasting results anyway!

Factor Four

Resistance Training

(or Building Your Body's Best Fat-burning Machinery)

When the time for their next session arrived he walked into the office differently, he had confidence in the way he held his body. He felt tighter-skinned, more energetic, and attractive. His shirt-sleeves had begun filling in and he even tightened his belt two notches! It was the belt he had used for a gauge to see if he was making progress—and he was! Although his weight had not dropped as much as he had hoped his body was feeling and looking better than he had expected. And the weights he was lifting, it was like he was back in High School. He loved the feeling of power! He was giddy to begin this next section of his training and although he knew it would be really hard, he welcomed it!

The trainer noticed the difference in his posture and smiled, knowing that he was beginning to understand and master the Factors of Fitness! "Welcome back, you are looking confident!" The trainer said as he led the man to the desk. "We are going to start at the desk today and cover some conceptual information before heading to the gym to exercise."

They sat down in their usual seats and the trainer pulled out a binder with his cards, a bucket of feathers, and a small stone. "Several weeks ago we talked about how important exercise is to fat loss and for maintaining it. If you recall, we talked about how when you increase your fat free mass you dramatically increase your metabolism and it helps you burn energy all day everyday. In fact, a 25-year study concluded that exercise combined with diet modification is the best way to lose fat and keep it off![38] We also discussed how cardio exercise does not stimulate muscle and bone growth like resistance exercise does, making the latter indispensable. Today we will move on to the Fourth Factor: resistance training. Now, when I say resistance training I include within that phrase the traditional weight lifting *and* flexibility and core training."

"In other words, weight lifting, stretching, and ab work? What's with the feathers and rock?" He asked.

"Before we get to the feathers and rock let me clarify that flexibility is more than stretching and that core training is more than working your 'abs'. Flexibility can be broken down into a couple categories: stretching and myofascial release. Stretching can be further broken down into static and dynamic stretching. Core training involves working your 'abs' as well as many other muscles connecting between your pelvis and spine or your pelvis and ribcage. We will go more in depth with each of these, but first let's get to the feathers!" He picked up the rock and the feathers. "Which weighs more this pound of feathers or this one pound rock?"

"I remember this from grade school. They are the same. They are both a pound." The man said sardonically.

"Right! Often in grade school when kids begin to grasp the concepts of mass and density, they begin the jokes about what weighs more—feathers or something heavy like this stone. The lesson for us today is about fat-free mass, fat, and their different densities. Because fat-free mass is more dense than fat it requires less space for the same weight."

---

[38] Miller WC, Kocaeja DM, & Hamilton EJ. A meta analysis of the past 25 yrs. of weight loss research using diet, exercise, or diet plus exercise intervention. *International Journal of Obesity.* 1997; 21: 941-47.

"English please!"

"What this means is that you could take your size ten pants and fit into them quicker if you lost ten pounds of fat but gained ten pounds of fat-free mass…"

"Because I might weigh more but would be smaller!"

"That's right! Let's move on to flexibility now!"

"I remember hearing or reading about some people now saying that stretching is not good for you and that it shouldn't be done, is that true?"

"No, but I do know what you are talking about. Back in 2008, a professor at the University of Nevada published a study in the *Journal of Strength and Conditioning Research.* The study demonstrated that muscles decrease performance if they are statically stretched prior to exercising because it causes neurological inhibition, which means the nervous system prevents full function in that area.[39] Static stretching can be thought of as the old gym stretches we used to do; like when we would bend over to touch our toes and hold the position for 20-30 seconds."

"Good; I hated doing those stretches!"

"Well, you will still need to do them—the research only showed that it decreased performance before exercise but it still is a good way to prevent injuries! From this and similar research they have found that the best method of stretching prior to exercise is a dynamic style; where you are moving the joints and muscles that will need to be used, but you are not holding the position. What we are doing with this is providing increased blood flow and heat to the muscles and joints that will be used during exercise.[40] Warm muscles and dilated blood vessels more efficiently do two important functions during exercise. First, they pull oxygen from the bloodstream better and second they more efficiently use stored energy from muscles. Both of

---

[39] www.nsca-jscr.org.

[40] www.nytimes.com/2008/11/02/sports/playmagazine/112pewarm.html?_r=0

these functions are significant contributors to exercise performance! Another important result of the warmed-up muscle is that it is far less likely to rip during extreme exercise! After exercising is when you should perform your static stretching because it will help improve flexibility but will not decrease performance!

We will use this type of stretching for the traditional overall increase in flexibility but also for corrective stretching. Corrective stretching is focusing static stretching on specific muscle groups to help decrease muscular imbalances."

"I think I get what you mean about muscle imbalances but just to be sure can you explain it a little more?"

"Sure. Our body is designed to move by muscles shortening. They are anchored at two points, usually on two different bones, spanning across a joint. When a muscle shortens it pulls those two points closer together, causing one of the bones to move. Here's the kicker—muscles can only move a bone one direction! For this reason we have an opposite muscle that shortens to return the bones to their original position." Seeing his sustained confusion the trainer rolled up his sleeve to mid-arm. "See my biceps here? Watch as a move my hand closer to my shoulder…do you see the muscle getting shorter? Now, I cannot use the biceps to move my hand away from my shoulder so I have to use the triceps on the back of the arm to do that. See how the biceps are elongating while my triceps are shortening? They work in concert with each other! Problems arise when one muscle in a pair is too tight because it does not allow the partner muscle to fully elongate. This is a self-perpetuating problem because the elongated muscle weakens over time and the shortened muscle tightens over time. Immediately the body begins to create compensatory strategies and these can become ingrained so deeply that we move and live in an altered way without ever knowing it. We use the wrong muscles for movements. When a muscle is in a semi-shortened position from an imbalance a phenomenon called <u>Synergistic</u> <u>Dominance</u> occurs. This is where the semi-shortened muscle does work that it should not be doing or it does more of the work than it should, taking a primary-mover role rather than a secondary-mover role. This keeps us from strengthening all the muscles we need to! When we do this we also wear out areas of joint prematurely. The probability of injury significantly increases!"

"Yeah, let's avoid that!"

"Right, I noticed that injuries were not on the goal list you gave me! You have what is the most common imbalance in our nation—a protracted shoulder girdle. Have you ever notices how your shoulder are rounded and slouch forward?"

"My Dad never let me forget it! He was always harping on me to sit up or stand up straight! To pull my shoulders back!"

"The imbalance is between the chest muscles, pectoralis major and minor, and a back muscle, the latissimus dorsi, muscles being too tight while the muscles between your shoulder blades, rhomboids and middle trapezius, being too weak. This imbalance is a result of gravity and lifestyle working against us every waking hour! Gravity is always pulling our shoulders down and forward and pretty much everything we do in life is in front of us. When we drive, sit at a desk, sit and watch TV, or type at a computer we shorten the chest muscles and lengthened the back muscles! Stand back up and relax your posture; I want to show you something." He waited until the man had relaxed into a comfortable position. "See how your thumbnails point towards the front of your hips? That is an indication of tight lats, or latissimus dorsi, which inserts at the front of the upper arm. As the muscle tightens it rotates the arm internally, which results in the thumbnail facing the side of the body. The tighter the lats are the more the thumbnails face the hips. When the lats are properly lengthened, the thumbnails face forward, are parallel, and would not intersect if lines were drawn from them."

The man looked at his arms and hands and saw what the trainer was talking about. "I see it! I totally understand what you are saying; cool!"

"Glad to see you understand! For us to correct this we will be doing stretches for your tight chest and Lat muscles while strengthening your weakened back muscles. And by 'we' I mean *you*." He said with a smile.

"Of course you do! If you could do it *for* people you would be rich!" Was the reply.

"If only! There is one more concept tied to flexibility that we need to cover and that is myofascial release. 'Myo' is Latin for muscle and 'fascial' means loose tissue. 'Myofascial' refers to the combination of these two materials as they occur within the body. Fascia is that white and silvery tissue that surrounds a steak but is not the fat. It is an intricate network of tissue that is interconnected from our head to our toes. In the muscles, it surrounds each muscle fiber, or cell, and each cell is bundled together with another layer of fascia. These bundles are again packaged and wrapped in fascia in larger bundles over and over until you have the actual full muscle. The fascia continues and at each end of the muscle and they are interwoven into a strong cord, which is a tendon. This material also surrounds bones, organs, blood vessels, and the underside of all your skin! The beauty of this system is that it holds us all together and allows things to adjust and adapt to changes in the body, allowing us to still function well. The facial network is much like a knit sweater. Have you ever had a knit sweater and gotten a snag in it?"

"Oh yeah, they are impossible to fix. The more you mess with it the more of a mess it becomes! ...And saying that, I get the point. If there is tightness in one spot of you body it can affect other areas because they are all connected!"

"Correct! In fact, I remember a story from one of my initial training certifications about a professional baseball player who was warned by the athletic trainers that his calves were too tight and that he needed to give extra attention to stretching them. He ignored this advice or did not fully follow it and near the end of the season he tore his rotator cuff, which is a group of muscles in the shoulder. Since everything is connected and his calves were too tight, his body had to change the mechanics of throwing from his knees to his shoulders. The new mechanics created a force that slowly destroyed his shoulder!"

"Oh, that's terrible! Why didn't he just do his stretches?"

"It was not necessarily that simple. The static and dynamic stretching that we have discussed will not address some flexibility issues. This guy easily could have developed an adhesion. An adhesion is a knot of fascia caused by a trauma. The layers of fascial tissue get 'glued' together during cellular reconstruction and no longer slide past each other and get bound together in a ball. The ball prevents full normal range of motion from the muscle. This causes all kinds of problems like decreased motion and the compensatory movements I told you about earlier. The static and dynamic stretches address flexibility primarily within the muscle cell and the tendon. The long muscle cells have special sections called muscle spindles that cause contraction when too much elongation is placed on a muscle; they prevent over stretching and tearing. There is another special cell, called the Golgi Tendon Organs, located next to the ends of the muscle fibers, at the beginning of the tendon. These cells regulate the muscle length according to tension on the muscle. They too prevent over stretching and tearing. So, neither of these actually address the fascial network or an adhesion! That baseball player may have been doing static and dynamic stretches but not fixing the problem!

To address an adhesion, pressure needs to be applied to literally break apart the layers of connective tissue. Once they have been separated they can slide past each other again. This is the type of thing that a massage therapist will do when you get one of those really painful massages where the therapist digs an elbow into a knot and presses on it! Have you seen those foam rollers around the gym?" He said pointing to a long cylindrical white foam form propped in the corner. After he nodded affirmatively the trainer continued, "We will use those to break up the adhesions that you have and keep you flexible!"

He showed the man how to locate adhesions by identifying tender spots in a muscle. Then he showed him how to position his body so that gravity was pushing the body weight against the adhesion to separate the layers. He instructed him in the rules for safety and effectiveness and gave him a card with the instructions:

<u>SELF MYOFASCIAL RELEASE:</u>

1. Roll towards your heart.

2. Never role over bones.

3. Never role over joints.

4. Hold on top of the adhesion until you feel a release and less pain.

5. Perform prior to exercises.

The man took the card and then inquired, "Why would you do this one before exercise?"

"Since this type of exercise does not trigger the neurological inhibition that static stretching triggers there should not be any decrease in exercise performance. It is a mechanical problem, not a neurological one. Let's go practice what you just learned!" He said standing up and indicating the doorway to the gym.

They entered the gym and after a short warm up he used the foam roller on his illiotibial (IT) band, hamstrings, and calves; all of which were riddled with tender spots. The pain was almost unbearable and he wanted to stop early several times but the thought of giving up in front of the trainer seemed more painful, so he pressed on and finished the task. Although he did not feel any different the trainer informed him that it was normal to feel that way and that, as with all flexibility training, it takes consistent effort for awhile before noticing improvements in his range of motion.

"Now that you have endured the pain of self myofascial release it is time to learn about your core musculature and how to properly train it." He followed the trainer over to a mat on the floor and turned to face a human anatomy poster that the trainer was standing next to. "Do you see these muscles that connect from the bottom of the ribcage down to the pelvis bones?" He said pointing at the midsection of the body.

"Yes. Those are the abs, right? I see the six muscles that make up your six-pack. I work these while doing crunches or sit-ups. This is an area I *really* want to focus on! I want to lose that stubborn belly fat and get rid of the beer belly!" He joked patting his belly.

"Now, I know that you are partially joking but how much I am not sure; so we are going to discuss spot reduction before going any further about the core! In the mid 80's the

University of Massachusetts conducted a study on the effects of site-specific exercise on the body-fat at those sites. This study lasted 27 days and the 13 subjects involved performed a rigorous abdominal exercise program—they were required to do a total of 5,000 sit-ups! That's over 185 sit-ups each and every day! Before the study began and after it ended, fat biopsies were taken from the subjects' abdomens, buttocks and upper backs. Contrary to what late-night infomercials and spot-reducing proponents would have you believe, the results of the study revealed that fat decreased similarly at all three sites! There was no extra fat loss for the area exercised![41] More recently, another study used at the University of Connecticut used a 12-week resistance program that only trained one side of the body and the results were the same—no difference in body fat between the trained side and the untrained side![42] There also have been studies conducted with professional tennis players who use one side of their body *far* more frequently than the other. These studies have also shown that spot-reduction is a myth! So, I know that you really want to lose the fat around your waist, hips, and butt; however, your body will take the fat from where it wants to and when it wants to. I have had clients lose fat like an ice cube melting—kind of all over at once, and I have had clients who lose it more in certain areas first. It is too soon to see what your body is going to do. But remember the First Law of Thermodynamics—if you create a deficit you will lose fat! Even if your body chooses to take it from your waist last, it will eventually have to take it from there!"

---

[41] www.acefitness.org/fitnessqanda/fitnessqanda_display.aspex?itemid=341 Retrieved 12/22/12.

[42] Kostek M, Pescatello L S, Seip R L, Angelopoulos T J, Clarkson P M, Gordon P M, Moyna N M, Visich P S, Zoeller R F, Thompson P D, Hoffman E P, Price T B. Subcutaneous fat alterations resulting from an upper-body resistance training program. *Medical Science Sports Exercise.* 2007 July; 39(7): 1177–1185. doi: 10.1249/mss.0b0138058a5cb

The man smiled, "I *was* half-joking you know! But that is all good to know; I still did have that little thought bouncing around that if I just did more crunches my abs would look great! You had just shown me the six-pack when I got us side-tracked."

"Yes. The muscle is called the rectus abdominus and it is one of over two-dozen muscles that comprise what we call the core. The thing I want you to note here is the direction of the muscle fibers. As we discussed during corrective stretching, muscles move bones by the shortening of muscle cells connected at two different bones. The rectus decreases the angle of spine, called <u>flexion</u>, by moving the ribcage and the pelvis closer together. This happens during a crunch when the ribcage is moved towards the pelvis but it also can happen when the pelvis is moved towards the ribcage. Notice that both exercises move *in* the direction of the muscle fibers! All exercises should do that to maximize their effectiveness. Now, look at these muscles along each side of the rectus. They intersect the rectus at an oblique angle, which is where they get their names—the obliques. These are the external obliques but you also have a set of internal obliques that are arranged in the opposite direction. The obliques' function is to help flex the spine *and* rotate it. The most common exercise for this is a side crunch or sit-up with rotation. Deeper than those layers is the innermost abdominal—the transverse abdominus, or TVA. This muscle has muscle fibers that run almost horizontally, parallel to the waistline of your pants. We will spend the most time discussing this latter one because you already have some information about working the more external muscles and because the TVA is the biggest culprit in low back injuries.[43]

---

[43] Teyhen DS, Miltenberger CE, Deiters HM, et al.. The use of ultrasound imaging of the abdominal drawing-in maneuver in subjects with low back pain. *Journal of Orthopedic Sports Physical Therapy. 2005* Jun;35(6). 346-55.

The challenge with our TVA is that it has been so neglected by our lifestyles that it loses the ability to contract when needed. When we sit, which is most of our lives, we are stretching the TVA muscle fibers. Just like the muscle imbalances we discussed during flexibility training, if the muscle is stretched it eventually loses strength. The TVA usually has become so weak that the more superficial abdominal and low back muscles usurp the nerve impulse and the TVA never does the job it was designed to do."

"The signal is stolen by other muscles? Sounds like that one syn thingy you mentioned earlier...."

"Synergistic Dominance! Right on, that's exactly what it is! Our bodies are so used to those external muscles doing the work they can no longer get the correct muscles to do it! Because of this we have three stages, or levels, of work to do with the TVA. The first stage is isolation. This stage is where you will be trying to reconnect the full nerve impulse with the TVA. You will notice that when you draw your belly-button in towards your spine that either your pelvis wants to rotate, because your rectus abdominus and lower back muscles are pulling on your pelvis, or that you suck in your waist by holding your breath, which is just elongating your waist—stretching it thinner! Once you are able to isolate the muscle again you can move to the second stage, integration. Integration is where you will begin to strengthen your TVA, similar to traditional weight training. When your TVA is strong enough you will move to the third and final stage—mobility. The mobility stage is where you will learn to properly stabilize your lower spine with your TVA during body movements.

Because of the wide variety of muscles used and their diverse locations it is important to perform core exercises in both prone and supine positions. A prone position is where you face the floor, like in a plank exercise. A supine position is where you face the ceiling, like in a bridge exercise." He went through the exercises with the man; giving praises, corrections, tips and advice as warranted.

"What's next?" He asked

"We need to establish some uniform terminology and concepts before continuing; that way we are having disciplined discourse and fully understand each other. The first thing that we will do is talk about program components. Exercise programming is tethered to the energy processes the body uses to produce movement. There are three energy systems your body uses: the aerobic, the glycolytic, and the ATP-PCr systems.[44] All three of these are always being used, just in varying proportions. A good exercise program considers a person's goals and matches it with the energy system that will best support change towards that goal. Do you know what aerobic means?"

The man shook his head yes, "It is exercise that uses oxygen; like running, biking, or swimming."

"That's correct, it means that the exercise relies on oxygen as its primary source of energy! The other two systems are what we call anaerobic, meaning that oxygen is not their primary source. Remember that our bodies use all three, just in differing degrees depending on the demands."

"What do you mean by demands? Like how much work is being done?"

"Partially, yes. The *amount* of work coupled with the *type* of work determines which energy system takes the lead role in energy production. The aerobic system requires far longer to produce energy than the other two systems; however, when it does produce energy

---

[44] Wilmore JH, Costill DL, Kenney WL. (2008) *Physiology of sport and exercise.* 4th ed. Champaign, IL: Human Kinetics. 50-55.

it produces more than *ten times* the energy of the next most productive system—the glycolytic!"

" So, activities that require smaller muscles working at a lower intensity can afford the time to use the aerobic system? But other activities that use bigger muscles at a higher intensity don't have the time to make enough stuff to do the work?" The man explained half to himself.

"Exactly right! For that reason we will need to closely monitor rest periods, tempo, and the order your exercises are performed in. Equally important are your sets and repetitions because resistance training is really like a cooking recipe. All of these are like ingredients we use for making certain foods. For example, a cake, cookie, and piecrust all use some of the same basic ingredients—time, temperature, flour, sugar, eggs, and a dash of salt! But, they all combine those ingredients in different amounts to produce different results. One creates a moist and soft cake, another a firm dense cookie, and the third a flaky, butter crust. Our bodies have the same diverse responses to resistance exercise! I have trained people to run marathons faster, focusing on their aerobic system. I have trained people to get massively muscular and body-build by focusing on the glycolytic system. I have improved power-lifters one rep max using the ATP-PCr system. Most relevant to you, I have trained people to lose fat by using all the systems in ways at different times to get that result. For your goal, we will initially use the glycolytic system to build fat-free mass because it is your body's best fat-burning machinery!"

"Remember, I don't want to get freaky-huge with veins popping out everywhere like a bodybuilder! I want to look lean, muscular, and athletic!" He protested.

"A reasonable fear, based on what you have seen in muscle magazines!" The trainer assured him, "But believe me when I say that normal men have little to fear from aggressive resistance training. You have neither the genetics nor the hormones to become 'freaky-huge', as you put it. The men you see on TV or in magazines with those physiques are using Factor Six!"

"I thought there were only five factors? What is factor six?" He puzzled aloud.

"There *are* only five factors of fitness for improved aesthetics *and* health. That is why I call steroid and drug use Factor Six! It is something you need to avoid to reach your goals of looking good and *being* healthy! The point is that those men are treating themselves with potentially damaging male hormones and drugs that stimulate muscle growth; unless you do that too you don't need to worry about looking that way!" The trainer said handing him a card that read:

Resistance Training:

Make muscles—your best fat burning machinery!

"Okay. What will my program be?" He conceded, knowing that the trainer would throw more studies at him if he protested.

The trainer smiled, knowing that the capitulation was good-natured and out of respect, "First we need to discuss proprioceptive demand, exercise selection, keeping constant tension on the muscle through the full range of motion, and proper form before we get into the specifics of your program.

Proprioception is your recognition of how your body relates to space. Proprioceptive demand is an exercise technique used to destabilize your body during exercise. Studies have shown that decreasing your stability increases the recruitment of muscle for the same exercise at the same level of intensity. For my graduate-level physiology course we had to do research projects and my group chose to use EMG (Electromyography) technology to test the results of those studies. We hooked the electrodes up to subjects' chest muscles on the right side and had them bench press the same dumbbell weight in four positions: lying on a stable bench and pressing dumbbells simultaneously with both arms, lying on a stability ball and pressing dumbbells with both arms, and lying on a stability ball and pressing with only the right arm. The EMG data showed a statistically significant increase in muscle activation at each level of destabilization; the stable bench pressing both arms used much less energy than the single arm press on the stability ball. This confirmed what I had read in other studies!"

"And for me, I can lift less weight and get more calorie burn by using less stable things to stand, sit, or lay on, right!" He asked proud of making the connection before being told.

"Exactly right! The general hierarchy of safest and least effective modes of exercise to most risky and effective is the following," The trainer said handing him a card:

HIERARCHY OF EXERCISES:

1. Machines

2. Pulleys

3. Barbell Free-weights

4. Dumbbell Free-weights

5. Dumbbells with destabilization

6. Single-sided dumbbells with destabilization

7. Single-sided dumbbells with destabilization and rotation

"This pyramid starts at the top with the most safe but least effective exercise modes. When you are capable of exercising at level seven make sure that the dumbbell you use crosses your midline when you rotate! This further destabilizes you and increases calorie burn through muscle activation. We will use this knowledge to maximize your time and efforts during workouts all the while reducing the risk of joint and soft-tissue injury! You will lose fat quicker and more safely! It is a win-win!" He told the man excitedly. "This principle is a pillar for your exercise selection when creating a resistance program!"

"But I thought you were going to set me up with a program!" The man protested feeling a bit overwhelmed.

"I *am* going to set you up with one but remember what I said back when we first met— my philosophy is to teach you how and why to do the right things so you *know* why you are successful. I want you to be able to create and revise programs for yourself when we are no longer meeting! Okay?

Let's get back to exercise selection; we need to pick the 'just-right' fit for your physical capabilities so that you get the most out of each and every rep. Essentially we will perform a risk/reward analysis to chose each exercise you will be doing."

The man cocked his head to the side, "In other words, you are going to see how dangerous an exercise is and if that level of danger is worth the benefits of that exercise? If there is a safer way to get the same results we will do that exercise instead, right?"

"Yes. Some benefits can be achieved in a variety of ways. Certain exercises may be more dangerous than others depending upon your individual abilities and anatomy."

"Why would my anatomy make a difference?"

"There could be too high a risk due to the muscle imbalances we discussed earlier or there could be something about the way your body was designed. Some people have tighter joints than other people and they can cause injury by performing certain exercises. A perfect example is the shoulder. Most people have tight enough shoulder joints that they cannot safely perform behind the neck exercises like lat pull-downs or shoulder presses that come behind the head. They have too little space under the collarbone for the motion to not grind one of the rotator cuff muscles between the collarbone bone and the top of the upper arm bone. This results in inflammation, which creates even less space and exacerbates the problem. Eventually, if left unchecked, the person will develop what is called Impingement Syndrome. This is painful and sets people back in their activities because it requires rest of the shoulder for a long time to let the inflammation subside before resuming activities that involve the shoulder. If he would have chosen a different exercise that worked the same muscles but did not close that joint and cause grinding; he would have been able to exercise without problems and reached his goals sooner!

Before we get to the specifics of your program we have a couple more concepts to discuss—how to lift with proper form. Proper form is keeping constant tension on the target muscles through the full range of motion. I will show you the proper range of motion for your exercises in the weight room but I want you to pay attention to the feel of your muscles as you are using them. If you feel them become slack at a point near the beginning or end of the lift, you have lost the tension! This can be a result of recruiting other muscles to do the work, or overstretching the muscle. When this happens, you want to regain the tension by focusing on the correct muscle or modifying your range of motion. If you are unable to do this, then it is time to finish your set. I do not want you having sloppy form to get a few more reps because the risk outweighs the reward!

The final concept to discuss is when you will finish your sets. Most people think that they lift the weight until they are in the rep range in their program and then they stop at that point; makes sense, right?"

"It seems to, but you wouldn't be asking if it did!" The man joked.

"True. It seems counterintuitive at first so hear me out before asking questions. The rep range within a program is designed to maximize one of those energy systems, right? Well, if a person stops before that energy system is exhausted then there will not be the stimulation to force an improvement. Remember way back when we discussed needing to force the body to make changes? This is exactly what we need to do here! I want you to choose a weight that allows you to fail within the rep range indicated. For your program I will have you performing 15-20 reps on most exercises. This means that you chose a weight that you can lift at least 15 times but no more than 20, even if you had to! If you chose a weight you could lift 25 times and you stop at 20 does your body need to improve?" The man nodded a 'no'. "Right, if your body can lift a weight 25 times and you stop at 20 the muscle has no reason to improve because it can already do what you are asking it to do! Conversely, if you chose too heavy a weight and can only lift it 10 times, then you will be focusing your body on the wrong energy system and not have the adaptations that you are looking to make."

"I...think I get it." He offered in the hope the trainer would clarify.

"Let me give you a more concrete example with numbers; maybe that will help. Let's say that you are doing a chest press for 3 sets of 10-12 reps with 90 seconds of rest between sets. Last week you finished the exercise doing 50 pounds 10 times. Since you were able to finish the exercise at 50 pounds on the third set (after depleting some energy each previous set) you should be able to press 50 pounds on your first set for 12 times. So, this week you do your first set at 50 pounds and press it 12 times. Good! You are in the right range! You have 90 seconds of rest and believe you could press the same weight 10 times, still keeping in your rep range. So, you perform it again and press it 10 times. Good! You are still in the right range! Knowing what you do about energy systems you realize that you will not be able to press the 50 pounds for 10 reps in your final set so you decrease the weight to 40 pounds. This time your press the weight 12 times. Good! You are still in your rep range! This is how a good exercise session should be—decreasing weight or number or reps to create the best stimulation possible!"

"What if the 40 pounds had been too light? Should I have kept pressing for…say 15 reps? or 20 reps?"

"Yes. You want to achieve muscular failure—not being able to move the weight with safe form through the full range of motion. If you keep going to failure you can assess where to adjust your weights for the next session of training! Otherwise you are just guessing…"

"And your results reflect when you are guessing!" He interjected.

"True! You are wise beyond your years! Let's go on to the gym and get started on your individual program now." The trainer said smiling. From a file on his desk he withdrew a two-page sheet of paper with the program on it and led him to the gym. "Here is your individualized program. Each day of the week is broken down into four categories, which is also their order of operation! You will begin with a warm up then move on to your core exercises. After completing your core exercises, you will perform your resistance exercises and then end the session with flexibility exercises. Let's go through them one day at a time, starting with Monday."

"Here is your warm-up for a Monday. You will begin each resistance session by riding the bike for 5 minutes to elevate your overall body temperature. After those 5 minutes your will do your dynamic stretch, which on Mondays are Ball flies. This stretch is where you lay supine on a ball and slowly perform light flies—like you are hugging something!" He watched as the trainer positioned himself on a ball and demonstrated proper form. He showed the man on the program sheet where the warm up section was, "Make sure that you always perform your 5 minutes on the bike *and* dynamic stretches prior to resistance training! This section shows you all the details of your daily dynamic stretches. Notice it has 30-40 reps written but I only did a few to demonstrate. Make sure that you follow what is written on the program! Now it's your turn!"

After looking at the program sheet the man did a set and was helped with proper form.

Body Part	Dynamic Stretch	Reps
Chest	Ball Flies	30-40

He then relocated them to the mat area and positioned himself on the ground by having his hands beneath his shoulders and his knees beneath his hips. "This is the position from which you will perform Mondays' core exercise. The key to this exercise is to activate the transverse abdominus (TVA). From this position you will rotate your pelvis as far back as you can, making a swayback, then rotate as far forward as you can, flattening the low back. Once you have found these two points you rotate the pelvis to the middle of those two extremes; we call this neutral spine. Once you are in neutral spine you want to keep your pelvis there throughout the exercise—don't let the exterior abs and low back pull it out of place! In neutral spine you will pull your belly button in towards your spine as far as possible and hold that contraction for a count of ten. I want you to actually count aloud to ten and then push out your belly as far as you can. Pay attention to two things. First, there should be no pelvic rotation; if there is then it is the result of your abs and low back trying to pull the belly button in rather than allowing the TVA to do it. Second, there should be no change in your speech or breathing throughout the count to ten. If you find yourself rushing at the end or your voice getting fainter then you are elongating your torso and holding your breath to pull the belly button in. These two things are not unusual but you need to focus on stopping them and using the TVA. It truly comes down to a mental focus to reconnect the brain to the right

muscle!"

Body Part	Core Exercise	Reps	Sets	Rest
Core: TVA	Quadruple Draw-in Maneuver	10	3	20s

The man knelt down in position and the trainer helped him focus on how to recognize

neutral spine. He referred to the program sheet, "I want you to do three sets of ten reps and to

rest twenty seconds between each set."

The man stopped him with and upraised hand. "What makes a rep for these? Am I only

holding it for 10 seconds total?"

"Good question. No, a repetition is constituted by pulling in the belly button, counting to

ten, then pushing out the belly button as far as possible. Make sure that you rest the twenty

seconds between each set so that you get the most out of each one." He helped him through

the exercise and he learned how to recognize synergistic dominance and when he was

holding his breath. He struggled to use the correct muscle and was reminded that it is

difficult to do and that it takes time to retrain the body, "You've been doing wrong for nearly

30 years, so do not expect to just change it over the course of a workout or even over the

course of a week's worth of workouts!"

They moved over to the weight machines and he instructed the man on how to adjust the

machines to the correct position. He discussed, then demonstrated proper form. "The most

important thing for you to remember, because you will rarely find this info in any magazine

you read, is to not move your arms more than about an inch past the plane of your back. This

means that you almost could do these exercises lying on the floor! If you had a one-inch bench you could properly perform these lifts with dumbbells while lying on that bench. When you set up your machines and their seat positions, you should have tension on your muscle just past that one-inch location. Setting it there allows you to lift off the weight at a point that is relatively harmless and when you lower the weight during each rep the weight plates will not touch the rest of the weights on the stack. If you hear 'clinking' after a rep you have gone too far and the weights have been lowered to the point of touching the rest of the stack. When the weights touch the rest of the stack, your muscles do not have to do any work because gravity is pulling the weights down unto the stack; you can hold the handle all day and not have to do any work for the weight to remain in place. This is how you keep constant tension on the muscle through the full range of motion! It is important to keep the tension constant so that you get the most out of every rep!" He took a card from his folder, "I will hold onto this for you until your workout is finished!"

Keep Constant Tension on the Muscles Through the Full Range of Motion!

"Okay, thanks." He said as he slid into the seat and adjusted it like he had instructed. As he performed the exercises the trainer corrected him and helped him reposition as needed.

Body Part	Resistance Exercise	Sets	Reps	Rest	Tempo
Chest	Machine Chest Press	4	15-20	60 seconds	1-1-1
Chest	Cable Flies	4	15-20	60 seconds	1-1-1
Chest	Low to High Cable Flies	4	15-20	60 seconds	1-1-1

After taking him through the exercises and making sure that his form was correct they relocated back to the mats and discussed the stretching routine for his cool down.

Body Part	Static Stretch	Sets	Time
Chest	Wall Chest	1 (B)	25-30 seconds
Lats	Ball Lat Stretch	1 (B)	25-30 seconds

After reviewing the sheet the man asked, "What's the (B) stand for?"

"That is an abbreviation for 'bilateral', which is the medical term for 'both sides'. Either way you want to remember it works for me; just make sure that what you do to one side you do to your other side when you see a (B)."

They went through the stretching exercises and then went back to the desk to set their appointment for the next day. It was not much of a work out because of all the education that took place but he could tell that when he came back to do it for real it would be a great one!

The Full Monday Program:

Body Part	Dynamic Stretch	Reps			
Chest	Ball Flies	30-40			

Body Part	Core Exercise	Reps	Sets	Rest	
Core: TVA	Quadruple Draw-in Maneuver	10	3	20s	

Body Part	Resistance Exercise	Sets	Reps	Rest	Tempo
Chest	Machine Chest Press	4	15-20	60 seconds	1/1/01
Chest	Cable Flies	4	15-20	60 seconds	1/1/01
Chest	Low to High Cable Flies	4	15-20	60 seconds	1/1/01

Body Part	Static Stretch	Sets	Time		
Chest	Wall Chest	1 (B)	25-30 seconds		
Lats	Ball Lat Stretch	1 (B)	25-30 seconds		

The next four days when they met the routine was the same. The trainer took him through the next day of his program and emphasized those areas that would typically be improperly performed. On Tuesday it was to get a good "pinch" between his shoulder blades when performing the seated row. "Most people allow their biceps to do most of the work and you never really get the back workout that you need. He also explained lever-arms and how the man could use his body to increase the difficulty of his sit-ups. "The further away a load is from the fulcrum (your point of movement) the more work that is required to move it. During a sit-up your fulcrum starts as your lower back and ends as your hips. Your arms' positions can increase the difficulty of the exercise by moving them further from your pelvis. The easiest position is with your hands by your hips, followed by your hands across your chest. To increase your resistance you would then put your hands behind your head. If you still needed increased resistance you would then straighten your arms behind past your head."

The Full Tuesday program:

Body Part	Dynamic Stretch	Reps			
Back	Blue Theraband Rows	30-40			

Body Part	Core Exercise	Reps	Body Part	Rest	
Core: Abs	Sit ups	25-35	Core: Abs	20s	

Body Part	Resistance Exercise	Sets	Body Part	Rest	Tempo
Back	Seated Rows	4	Back	60 seconds	1-1-1
Back	Lat Pull Downs	4	Back	60 seconds	1-1-1
Back	Dumbbell Shrugs	4	Back	60 seconds	1-1-1

Body Part	Static Stretch	Sets	Body Part		
Back	Trapezius Stretch	1 (B)	Back		
Back	Ball Lat Stretch	1 (B)	Back		

Whenever he would let the weights touch the stack, go too far past in his range of motion, or use the wrong muscles to move the weight; the trainer pulled out his card saying, "Remember!"

> # Keep Constant Tension on the Muscles Through the Full Range of Motion!

Wednesday was a much needed and earned day off. He still did his cardio routine and ate well, but he was told to let his joints and tendons recuperate from the intense training with weights. Although he was beginning to become more comfortable at the gym and almost welcomed his resistance sessions he still welcomed this time to allow his body to rest and heal.

Thursday was business as usual. The trainer took him through the next day of his program and emphasized those areas that would typically be improperly performed. It was not swinging the arms when performing his biceps curls. "If your elbow is coming forward a lot then you are using your front shoulder muscles to move the weight. This means that you have not done this!" He said producing his card.

> # Keep Constant Tension on the Muscles Through the Full Range of Motion!

"The name triceps literally means 'three heads' in Latin, and your upper-arm's relation to your torso affects which of the three heads is doing most of the work. When your upper arm is parallel to your torso, two of the triceps do most of the work. When your upper arm is perpendicular to your torso, the third muscle assumes more of the work and those other two do not work as much."

"I don't get it. Why is there a difference; they still do the same thing?" He inquired.

"Good question. The muscle heads all connect at one end at the elbow but at the other end two of them connect at the upper arm bone whereas the third connects at the shoulder blade. This changes the length-tension relationship. This is the relationship of a muscle's connection points and the muscle's length in certain positions. Certain positions allow more muscle tissue to pull itself shorter, which produces more power. With the triceps, the section of the muscle that connects to the shoulder blade is in its best position to contract when the arm is perpendicular to the torso. As you progress we will switch your triceps' exercises to have some in each position! One caution with the triceps is that keeping tension on them requires you keep a 90-degree or more bend at the elbow. Your arm should never be bent more than the capitol letter 'L' shape! When you go past that L–shape, you overstretch the muscles and lose…"

"The tension on it; got it!" He said with a smile. "I think you really want to have me remember that!"

"It is one of the cornerstones of a safe and effective resistance program. Whether you are using bands, machines, or free-weights there must be constant tension on the muscle through the full range of motion for you to get the most out the exercise!"

The full Thursday program:

Body Part	Dynamic Stretch	Reps	
Arms	Blue Theraband curls	30-40	

Body Part	Core Exercise	Reps	Body Part
Core: TVA	Supermans	20	3

Body Part	Resistance Exercise	Sets	Body Part
Arms	Dumbbell Biceps Curls	4	15-20
Arms	Triceps Pulley Pushdowns	4	15-20
Arms	Machine Shoulder Press	4	15-20

Body Part	Static Stretch	Sets	Body Part
Arms	Overhead Triceps Stretch	1 (B)	25-30 seconds
Arms	Cross-Chest Delt Stretch	1 (B)	25-30 seconds

Friday the trainer took him through the final day of his program and again emphasized those areas that would typically be improperly performed. He had learned so much but he was particularly excited about today's lesson because it was on some of his trouble areas—he hated working his legs! He knew now that there was no such thing as spot reduction, but he did not care because it made him *feel* like things were getting done!

"There are three main safety rules that we are going to start with today. I want to make sure that you are as safe as possible during your transformation! First, never let your knees go past your toes in the frontal plane. When this happens, your knee joint gets pulled apart and you increase the chances of serious injury!"

The man stopped him with an upraised hand, "What is the frontal plane?"

"The <u>frontal plane</u> is a term for the plane of movement parallel with the front of your body. This plane divides your body into front and back sections. When you stand squared-up to the front of a mirror, both what you see of yourself and the mirror are in the frontal plane."

"I think I get it. If I were lying in a bathtub, the water would represent the frontal plane. As the water drained, the frontal plane would still be the surface of the water but it would change; at each point the water surrounded my body it would be the frontal plane, right?"

"Correct! When you are performing lunges and leg presses you do *not* want your toes to go past the frontal plane where your knees are. Think about if you were standing at a wall with your toes up against it. When you went into your movement your knees would never hit the wall your toes were touching.

The second safety rule for you is to maintain alignment of your hips, knees, and ankles. Stand with your feet directly beneath your knees and your knees directly beneath your hips. This is the alignment you need to maintain during you exercises. If you feel unsafe during your lunges then widen your stance as little as possible so that you can keep as close to this alignment as possible!

The final safety rule for your legs is about the proper range of motion. You do not want to allow your pelvis to move at the end of any leg exercise movement. This takes the tension off the proper muscles and is very dangerous for the lower back. The point where you feel your pelvis rotate means that you have gone too deep for the exercise range! Find this point without any weight during the exercise movement, and then always stop just short of that point during each repetition. This will save your back and get you the best lower-body workout!

The full Friday program:

Body Part	Dynamic Stretch	Reps	Body Part
Thighs	Walking lunges	30-40	
Body Part	**Core Exercise**	**Reps**	**Body Part**
Core	Supine ball curls	10	3
Body Part	**Resistance Exercise**	**Sets**	**Body Part**
Thighs	Leg Press	4	15-20
Thighs	Leg Curls	4	15-20
Thighs	Leg Extensions	4	15-20
Legs	Standing Calf Raises	4	15-20
Body Part	**Static Stretch**	**Sets**	**Body Part**
Thighs	Modified Hurdler	1 (B)	25-30 seconds
Thighs	Quad	1 (B)	25-30 seconds
Thighs	90/90	1 (B)	25-30 seconds
Legs	Wall Calf	1 (B)	25-30 seconds

The next few weeks consisted of exercising more with less discussion, and the man felt it everywhere in his body! He was sore in places that he did not know he had muscles. The trainer informed him that this was normal and that there was nothing to worry about unless the pain lasted for more than three or four days. He found that after two days the pain usually peaked and always was gone by the fourth day.

Although he weighed more than in the past, he was losing inches off his waist and felt tighter everywhere. Nearly as satisfying was the fact that there were fewer and fewer times during their workouts when the trainer pulled out the card saying, "Remember!"

Keep Constant Tension on the Muscles Through the Full Range of Motion!

Concerned about something he heard at work, the man asked the Trainer, "Don't I need to worry about creating too large a caloric deficit and causing myself to go into 'starvation mode' and it affecting my results?"

"What do you know about this mode?" Was the response.

"I heard some people at work talking about a mode your body gets into when it is worked too hard and in too big a caloric deficit. They said that it causes your body to shut down metabolic processes and you stop losing fat. I looked it up online and found the same information there; I don't want it to stop! I love what my body is turning into!"

"Before I answer your question, have you noticed the change in your language and thought processes? You are using the language of a Master of the Five Factors of Fitness!

This is a significant milestone in your journey to health and fitness! Congratulations! Now, let's discuss the facts about this 'mode.' Research has shown there is a 3-7% decrease in metabolism when a person is in a severe deficit.[45] Remember that pesky Law of physics we learned when we first met? It *still* applies because it *always* applies! Even when a person has a decrease in metabolism if she is in a deficit then the body must lose weight! A good caloric deficit will be at least more than 10% of a person's metabolism, so even if there were a 7% decrease, the person would still be losing fat at a 3% rate! Does that answer your question? As for the Internet and finding the same information there, the Internet is not regulated for truth. Anything can be written there without a shred of truth or evidence for it. You must check their sources carefully to see if there is evidence behind what they are saying. There was a point in history when the majority of Europe believed the Earth to be flat. Their belief did not make it so—no matter how many of them there were!" He said pulling out his binder and jotting down a note. "Now I have to make another card! Thanks!"

"My pleasure!" The man said with a smile, inwardly and outwardly.

"Speaking of cards—here is your next one." The trainer said pulling a card from the binder. "You are ready to master the final factor—although you have started on it without even being aware of it! Next time we meet, we will discuss social supports and how to use them for sustained success!"

---

[45] www.dotfit.com/content-5435.html?utm_source=iContact&utm_medium=email&utm_campaign=B2B%20Prospects&utm_content=

FACTOR FOUR

Resistance Training:

- Stretch before and after your workout.

- Fat Free Mass is your best fat-burning Machinery.

- There is no spot reduction!

- Use the right recipe!

- Keep constant tension on the muscle through the full range of

  motion!

- Congratulations! You have mastered the Fourth Factor!

He took the card with a smile. After quickly perusing it, he placed it with his now large collection of cards and headed out the door. Things were falling into place!

Factor Five

Social Support

(or You'll Quit on Yourself Before You'll Quit on Someone Else)

As the time for the next session drew near the man considered whether or not to meet with the trainer. He was doing so well; he was getting compliments at work, sleeping better, lifting more weights, running longer distances, and looking fantastic in the mirror! Then it happened—he had a long day at work, ate poorly, and skipped his workout! How could this happen? After all he had learned and now knew! The next day he was disappointed in himself and moped around, had an okay workout, and ate all right. That's when he realized that there must be something missing and the trainer knew exactly what it was. He would go see him and finish the training. He was only a Master of Four Factors and that was not enough to get him the permanent lifestyle change he craved. He still needed to become a Master of the *Five* Factors of Fitness! He called the trainer and set another appointment.

When he entered the room for their appointment he still had the confident, self-assured presence from the past but this time it was tempered by the knowledge that success never comes easy because it is a daily decision for health and fitness. He had a renewed desire to learn about the Fifth Factor and was excited to learn the final piece of information! He was quite surprised to see the trainer's chair empty at his desk, which was cleared off. He had never been late for a session. In fact, he was always waiting and prepared, often with an elaborate set up for effect! Five minutes passed, then ten. Now he was really beginning to worry. Did he write down the wrong date or time? What if the trainer had been hurt? What if the man did not learn the Fifth Factor?

At precisely ten minutes after their set appointment the trainer entered the room, from the main entrance. The man turned and saw him then jumped up saying' "Are you all right? I was beginning to worry that something had happened to you!"

"I was giving you time to feel what it is like to be on your own without the support that you have been using and come to expect." He said as he seated himself at the desk. "The time is coming when you will be a Master of the Five Factors of Fitness and your final lesson is about how to recognize and utilize social resources to help you stay successful. Last time we spoke I told you that you had already started on this Factor; I was referring to me! I have been a social support for you in your quest for health and fitness! It is time to expand your base of social support because our time together is coming to an end. You will need other people and organizations in place to provide you with the encouragement and accountability you have been getting from me. Here is your first lesson about social support." He handed him a card that had written on it:

> You Will Quit On Yourself Before You Will Quit On
>
> Others!

"It is part of human nature that we always want to present the best of ourselves to other people. If you have other people who know your fitness goals then you are more likely to follow through with any changes that you have told them about! This is a primary reason for the success with 12-step programs for alcohol and drug recovery groups. When a person is around others who will be checking in with them regularly, that person has an additional incentive to accomplish those tasks. We do not like letting other people down! In fact, studies have shown that even making a commitment to a pet increases the likelihood of fat loss![46]

You have done some amazing things over the course of our time together and I know that there were times when you would not have come in and exercised if I was not going to ask you about how it went the next day. I also know that there were times when you would not have eaten the same way had I not been meeting with you a few days later."

The man nodded his head, knowing it to be true. "That's true. But where will I find another person to help me do things right?" He did not like where this conversation was headed.

"That is what Factor Five is all about—helping you identify possible supports. Some you already have around you and in your life, but others will need to be introduced into your life. You will need to learn how to use the supports already in your life and how to incorporate the new ones. Let's figure out the supports you already have in your life so that we can strategize how to best use them! Once we are finished with that we will move on to supports that you don't, but could, have!"

The man agreed that it sounded good and they talked about all the supports he already had in his life. He wrote a list that included his:

---

[46] Kushner RF, Blatner DJ, Jewell DE, Rudloff K. The PPET Study: people and pets exercising together. *Obesity.* 2006; 14:1762-1770.

- Church

- Family

- Wife

- Friends

- Pet dog

- Internet

They formulated a set of strategies of when to best use each of these sources. The man

decided that his church would be a good support for when he felt down on himself and had a

bad day at work. His family would be a good resource for telling his goals to, so that he

could be kept accountable. His wife would be a good support for the day-to-day routine of

exercise and health eating. The Internet was a good resource for those times when he needed

more information to make changes in his program or look up a new exercise. He would make

a commitment to jogging his dog each day.

Next they researched local support groups for weight loss and picked out a couple that

seemed to fit best with his schedule and needs. They developed a plan for his to visit each

one, talk with members, and decide which he would start attending. With his plan in place he

stood to leave, feeling that he had that last extra piece that would make all the difference! He

did not know why, but he had felt as though he had to do it all on his own. It was reassuring

to know that there were other people and things that would be there for him!

The trainer stopped him, and as he handed him a final card said, "Remember, we are

more than just our bodies, but we *are* our bodies too! Do not be ashamed for taking the best

care of yourself!"

FACTOR FIVE

Social Support:

- You Will Quit On Yourself Before You Will Quit On Others!

- Do cardio classes or exercise with a friend!

- Find a weight loss group to attend!

- Use your computer!

- Congratulations! You are now a Master of the Five Factors of Fitness!

Conclusion

The man took the knowledge he had acquired and applied it daily. He knew why he had made changes and how to make other changes! He felt how he had heard a fit person would feel and it was a wonderful new experienced. When he looked at himself in a mirror while lifting weights he saw the person he had always known was in there—handsome, athletic, healthy, confident, and strong. He often felt like there was nothing he could *not* do, which he knew was not true but it was a great feeling nonetheless! He liked the way other people saw him now, not as another overweight-could-be-handsome person but as a handsome person! He always remembered the conversation that he had with the trainer about how we *are* our bodies; and he smiled. He had always known that, but now he *felt* it too! The man was no longer a "young" man but he felt better than he had in his prime! He was more energetic, slept more soundly, and liked himself more than ever before! It was as if a whole new world had been opened up to him. He was the master of his body and that mastery allowed him to do things that he only hoped and dreamed for in the past.

First, he decided to run a marathon. He changed his eating and exercising programs to allow for this goal. It was awkward at first…and time-consuming! Pulling out all the cards he had earned and using the knowledge that he had learned, he was able to put together a program that he *knew* would get him to his goal of running a marathon, if he followed it. With the help of his support systems, he followed through with the program and ran a marathon. Although his time was over four hours he was content to finish the race and hung his 'participation medal' in a prominent location. However, he realized that regularly pushing his body that much would have negative consequences on his bones and joints. Having accomplished that goal he wanted to move on to a different pursuit—this time related to aesthetics.

He decided to enter a physique competition since he did not like the unnatural veiny-looking bodybuilder appearance! He once again pulled out his cards and created a program to sculpt his body and he hired a posing coach to teach him how to present his body in the best possible form. Through months of intense discipline and sacrifice, he changed his body into a Greek god-like body and won his age category. However, he realized that the things he had to do to reach that look were extremely unhealthy and the results very short-lived! Within a week he was back to his pre-contest appearance. Having accomplished that goal he decided to find a point of contentment between the contest body and his 'off-season' body with conditioning between the marathon-level and 'off-season' level. He found his happy medium and settled into a rhythm of successful, healthy living!

One day at work while eating lunch in the break room a newly hired coworker was lamenting the failure of his New Year's resolution. The coworker was telling how he could not lose fat, that he had tried every diet, that his body was just supposed to be fat, and he should just give up!

The man reached into his wallet and pulled out a card, "Brother, don't do that! You can do it—anyone can! You just need to master the Five Factors of Fitness and you *will* get what you want."

The coworker replied, "That's easy for you to say, you are in good shape!"

The man looked him squarely in the eye and said, "Exactly. But I wasn't always this way. If you're serious about change, call this guy's number and he'll help."

Bibliography

Abidov T, Grachev SV, Klimenov AL, Kalynzhih OV. Effects of Rhododendron caucasicum extract on body weight and dietary lipid absorption in obese patients: A double-blind placebo controlled clinical study. Final Report: Russian Ministry of Health; Grant: No: 03-122-1997; Clinical Study Study; Project No: 0101-1997/ 8pp.

Ames BN. Low micronutrient intake may accelerate the degenerative diseases of aging through allocation of scarce micronutrients by triage. *Proc Natl Acad Sci* U S A. 2006 Nov 21;103(47). Epub 2006 Nov 13. Review.

Baker, RC, Kirshenbaum DS. Weight control during the holidays: Highly consistent self-monitoring as a potentially useful coping mechanism. *Health Psychology.* 1998; 17.

Cecrle, W E. *The psychology and spirituality of overeating and obesity in the US.* (2010) Cyclopean Pheonix and William E. Cecrle Publishing. Amazon.com

Comb GF. The vitamins, fundamental aspects in nutrition and health. Second Edition. San Diego: Academic Press; 1998.

Dollahite J, Franklin D, McNew R. Problems encountered in meeting the Recommended Dietary Allowances for menus designed according to the Dietary Guidelines for Americans. *Journal of the American Dietetic Association.* 1995; 95

Dulloo AG, Antic V, Montani JP. Ectopic fat stores: housekeepers that can overspill into weapons of lean body mass destruction. *International Journal of Obesity Related Metabolic Disorders.* 2004 Dec;28 Suppl 4.

Elia, M. Organ tissue contribution to metabolic rate. In: Energy Metabolism: Tissue Determinants and Cellular Corollaries, edited by J.M. Kinney. New York: Raven © 1992

Heynsfield SB, van Mierlo CA, van der Knaap HC, Heo M, Frier HI. Weight management using a meal replacement strategy. Meta and pooling analysis from six studies. *International Journal of Obesity Related Disorders.* (2003) May, 27 (5): 537-49.

Hill AM, Buckley JD, Murphy KJ, Howe PR: Combining fish-oil supplements with regular aerobic exercise improves body composition and cardiovascular disease risk factors. *American Journal of Clinical Nutrition* 2007 , 85.

http://fpwr.org/about-prader-willi-syndrome

Irwin, T. New Dietary Guidelines from the American Diabetes Association. *Diabetes Care.* 2002;25.

Jiang J, Torok N. Nonalcoholic steatohepatitis and the metabolic syndrome. *Metabolic Syndrome Related Disorders.* 2008 Spring;6(1):1-7. Review.

Kant AK. Reported consumption of low-nutrient-density foods by American children and adolescents: nutritional and health correlates, NHANES III, 1988 to 1994. *Archive of Pediatric Adolescent Medicine.* 2003 Aug;157(8).

Krebs-Smith SM, Guenther PM, Subar AF, Kirkpatrick SI, Dodd KW. Americans do not meet federal dietary recommendations. *Journal of Nutrition.* 2010 Oct;140(10):1832-8. Epub 2010 Aug 11.

Kostek M, Pescatello L S, Seip R L, Angelopoulos T J, Clarkson P M, Gordon P M, Moyna N M, Visich P S, Zoeller R F, Thompson P D, Hoffman E P, Price T B. Subcutaneous fat alterations resulting from an upper-body resistance training program. *Medical Science Sports Exercise.* 2007 July; 39(7): 1177–1185. doi: 10.1249/mss.0b0138058a5cb

Kushner RF, Blatner DJ, Jewell DE, Rudloff K. The PPET Study: people and pets exercising together. *Obesity.* 2006; 14:1762-1770.

Marra MV, Boyar AP. Position of the American Dietetic Association: nutrient supplementation. *Journal of the American Dietitians Association.* 2009 Dec;109(12).

Miller WC, Kocaeja DM, & Hamilton EJ. A meta analysis of the past 25 yrs. of weight loss research using diet, exercise, or diet plus exercise intervention. *International Journal of Obesity.* 1997; 21.

Phelan S, Wyatt HR, Hill JO, et al. *Obesity.* 2006.

Rolls BJ, Morris EL, Roe LS. Portion size of food affects energy intake in normal-weight and overweight men and women. *American Journal of Clinical Nutrition.* 2002.

Shils ME, Vernon RY. Modern Nutrition in health and disease. 7th edition. Philadelphia PA: Lea and Febiger;1988.

Shultz LO, et al. (2006). Effects of traditional and western environments on prevalence of type 2 diabetes in Pima Indians in Mexico and the U.S., *Diabetes Care.* 29.

Teyhen DS, Miltenberger CE, Deiters HM, et al.. The use of ultrasound imaging of the abdominal drawing-in maneuver in subjects with low back pain. *Journal of Orthopedic Sports Physical Therapy.* *2005* Jun;35(6).

Thorsdottir I, Tomasson H, Gunnarsdottir I, Gisladottir E, Kiely M, Parra MD, Bandarra NM, Schaafsma G, Martinez JA: Randomized trial of weight-loss-diets for young adults varying in fish and fish oil content. *International Journal of Obesity* (Lond) 2007, 31.

Wilmore JH, Costill DL, Kenney WL. (2008) *Physiology of sport and exercise.* 4th ed. Champaign, IL: Human Kinetics.

Wing RR, Hill JO. *Annual Review of Nutrition.* 2001; 21.

www.acefitness.org/fitnessqanda/fitnessqanda_display.aspex?itemid=341

www.americanheart.org

www.dotfit.com/content-3657.html

www.dotfit.com/content-1453.html

www.dotfit.com/content-5435.html?utm_source=iContact&utm_medium=email&utm_campaign=B2B%20Pro spects&utm_content=

www.epa.gov/risk_assessment/glossary.htm

www.fda.gov/food/DietarySupplements/default.htm

www.fda.gov/food/DietarySupplements/GuidanceComplianceRegulatoryInformation/Regula tionsLaws/ucm173996.htm

www.medical-dictionary.thefreedictionary.com/Fatty+Liver+Syndrome

www.medical-dictionary.thefreedictionary.com/triage

www.nsca-jscr.org.

www.nytimes.com/2008/11/02/sports/playmagazine/112pewarm.html?_r=0

www.siumed.edu/mic/research/nutrient/gi42sg.html

Glossary

Aerobic System: Also known as the Oxidative System, this system produces a 37-39 ATP net gain following its metabolic process and can indefinitely replace ATP via respiration. Example: It is the primary system used to run a race 400m or further.

ATP-PCr System: This system relies on readily available ATP stored within the working cells and has 3-15 seconds output. Example: It is the primary system used to run a race of 100m or less.

Collarbone: Also known as the clavicle it is located at both sides of the top of the ribcage, connecting to the breastbone/sternum.

Concentric: The part of an exercise when the primary muscle is shortening under tension. Example: During a biceps curl when the weight is being pulled towards the shoulder.

Dumbbell: a short, single handed weight used for resistance training; typically a bar handle with equal weight attached to each end. Example: a 10-pound weight on both sides of a 5-pound handle; making a 25-pound dumbbell.

Eccentric: The part of an exercise when the primary muscle is lengthening under tension. Example: During a bicep curl when the weight is being lowered away from the shoulder.

End Range: The point of maximal contraction during an exercise. Example: During a biceps curl when the weight has reached the top of the movement arc but has not begun its descent and.

First Law of Thermodynamics: Energy only can be changed from one form to another; not created or destroyed. Example: Rubbing your hands together will generate heat on your palms. Although it seems to be creating energy, it is not. The work from your muscles uses the chemical energy of your body, changes it to work energy in your muscles, and then into friction energy in your skin, expressed as heat. What actually happened is you've moved energy from your body through your muscles and into your hands.

Flexion: Decreasing the angle of a joint. Example: Bending the elbow flexes it.

Frontal Plane: The plane that separates a body into front and back sections. This plane can describe any location inside or outside of the body. Example: If you are standing with your toes against the wall then the wall would represent the frontal plane.

Glycolytic System: This system produces a 2-3 ATP net gain following its metabolic process and has 120 seconds of output prior to depletion. Example: It is the primary system used to run a race between 100m and 400m.

Law of Gravity: All objects in the universe pull on each other, the object with more mass wins the tug-of-war. On earth everything is pulled to the center of the planet. Example: You drop a ball and it is pulled towards the center of the earth until something stops it.

Length-Tension Relationship: The relationship between the length of a muscle and its ability to contract with force at that length. There is a point at which a shortened muscle loses strength and then cannot further shorten, called active insufficiency. There is another point the opposite direction at which a lengthened muscle loses strength and then cannot further lengthen, called passive insufficiency. Example: The biceps are actively insufficient when they are fully contracted and the hand is brought to the front of the shoulder. The biceps are passively insufficient when they are stretched by a fully straightened arm.

Neutral spine: The midpoint between the two extreme end range points of pelvic rotation.

Range of Motion (ROM): The distance a body part moves from start to finish. There are different types of ROM: such as anatomical and exercise. This book is referencing the exercise ROM.

Repetitions (reps): The number of times a movement is performed. Example: Lifting a weight once is a single rep; lifting a weight ten times is ten reps.

Rest periods: The amount of time waited between exercise sets. Example: Performing a set then resting 60 seconds before the next set is a rest period of 60 seconds.

Tempo: The speed at which a repetition is performed. It is reported in the concentric-end range-eccentric format. Example: During a biceps curl taking 1 second to raise the weight to the top of the range of motion, not pausing at the top, and taking 1 second to lower the weight to its start position is a tempo of 1-0-1.

Sets: A group of repetitions. Example: Performing ten reps then resting is a single set; performing ten reps, resting, then performing ten reps again is two sets.

Stability ball: A rubber, air-filled ball that is used for sitting, stretching, therapy, or exercises. Example: The 45cm, 55cm, and 65cm diameter balls seen in most gyms and therapy clinics.

Supine: Lying on your back. Example: Lying back on an exam table with your face to the ceiling.

Superficial: The layer of the body closer to the external environment in relation to a different body part. Example: The skin is more superficial than the muscles, which are more superficial than the bones.

Synergistic Dominance: Muscle(s) that are not designed to move a joint take over for the muscles that were designed to move that joint. Example: The elbow traveling forward during a biceps curl because the deltoid usurps some of the nerve impulse.

Prone: Lying on your stomach. Example: Lying on a massage table while the massage therapist works on your back.

Proprioception: Your body's awareness of itself in space. Example: Knowing that you are slouching while reading this book but without seeing your posture in a mirror.